Structure and Function of Antibodies

Edited by

L. E. Glynn and M. W. Steward
Canadian Red Cross Memorial Hospital,
Taplow, Bucks.
and
London School of Hygiene and Tropical Medicine
London

JOHN WILEY AND SONS

Chichester · New York · Brisbane · Toronto

British Library Cataloguing in Publication Data:

Structure and function of antibodies.
  1. Antigens and antibodies
  I. Glynn, Leonard Eleazar
  II. Steward, M. W.   III. Immunochemistry
  574.2'92   QR186.5   80-41379

ISBN 0 471 27917 X

Printed and bound in Great Britain
at The Pitman Press, Bath

List of Contributors

D. BEALE — Agricultural Research Council, Institute of Animal Physiology, Babraham, Cambridge, CB2 4AT, UK

A. FEINSTEIN — Agricultural Research Council, Institute of Animal Physiology, Babraham, Cambridge, CB2 4AT, UK

W. H. KONIGSBERG — Yale University School of Medicine, New Haven, Connecticut 16510, USA

F. F. RICHARDS — Yale University School of Medicine, New Haven, Connecticut 16510, USA

R. W. ROSENSTEIN — Yale University School of Medicine, New Haven, Connecticut 16510, USA

M. W. STEWARD — Division of Immunology, Kennedy Institute of Rheumatology, London W6 7DW, UK; now at: London School of Hygiene, Keppel Street, London WC1E 7HT, UK

M. W. TURNER — Department of Immunology, Institute of Child Health, Guildford Street, London WC1N 1EH, UK

J. M. VARGA — Yale University School of Medicine, New Haven, Connecticut 16510, USA

Contents

First published as Chapters 1, 2, 7, and 8 in *Immunochemistry: An Advanced Textbook*, edited by
L. E. Glynn and M. W. Steward. © 1977 by John Wiley and Sons Ltd.

Preface

The subject of immunochemistry owes much to the pioneering work of Paul Ehrlich but it was the physical chemist Arrhenius (1907) who first coined the word 'Immunochemistry' to describe:

> the chemical reactions of substances that are produced by the injection of foreign substances into the blood of animals (i.e. by immunization) and that the substances with which these products react as proteins and ferments are to be considered with respect to their chemical properties.

Much of the field of immunochemistry still has as its central theme the study of the chemistry of antibodies and antigens and their interaction. Since the time of Ehrlich and Arrhenius, knowledge of the structure and function of antibodies has expanded considerably and the four chapters of this book contain a comprehensive survey of current understanding of what is now well-recognized as probably the most complex and polyfunctional group of proteins known.

The book will be of particular value to undergraduates and postgraduates in both science and medical faculties interested in modern immunology and for research workers in immunologically oriented disciplines who wish to be acquainted with work in fields other than their own.

CHAPTER 1

Structure and Function of Immunoglobulins

M. W. Turner

1 GENERAL INTRODUCTION

Immunoglobulins are a family of structurally related proteins which mediate circulating antibody responses. There are five major classes of protein in most

Table 1 Human immunoglobulins

Present nomenclature	Abbreviation	Previous nomenclature
Immunoglobulin G	IgG	γ-G globulin, 7 S γ-globulin
Immunoglobulin A	IgA	γ-A globulin, β_2A-globulin
Immunoglobulin M	IgM	γ-M globulin, 19 S γ-globulin
Immunoglobulin D	IgD	
Immunoglobulin E	IgE	reagin, IgND

higher mammals although when the name immunoglobulin (Ig) was proposed by Heremans (1959) only three classes were known, namely IgG, IgA, and IgM. To these have now been added the classes IgD and IgE. Table 1 gives the present nomenclature recommended by WHO*.

Immunoglobulins are the products of lymphoid cells, particularly plasma cells, which synthesize large quantities of these proteins (see Chapter 4). Most immunoglobulin molecules produced by these cells are found in the serum and secretions of the body and are responsible for the humoral immune response. In addition, a small proportion of immunoglobulin molecules become firmly bound to the surface membranes of lymphocytes and macrophages and may function as antigen receptors, thus playing a role in implementing cell-mediated immunity.

The physicochemical heterogeneity of antibodies has been recognized for nearly 40 years and was a major problem in early structural investigations. However, in the mouse, rat, and man, pathological proteins occur known as myeloma proteins which are structurally homogeneous immunoglobulins produced by neoplastic plasma cells. Each of these proteins is thought to represent an overproduction of a single 'normal' immunoglobulin molecule, and in many cases sufficient protein has been isolated from serum to permit full immuno-chemical characterization. In the absence of myeloma proteins, such investigations would be almost impossible for the quantitatively unimportant IgD and IgE classes. ·

This chapter will attempt to provide a selective review of our present knowledge of the immunoglobulins. The emphasis will be largely on the human system but some information for other species will be included also, especially when notable differences occur. For convenience, the chapter is divided into a section dealing with general aspects of structure and a section devoted to the structural basis for effector or adjunctive functions such as complement fixation and interactions with membranes. The close relationships between primary structure and conformation are covered in Chapter 8 which should be considered conjointly with the present review.

* This and other aspects of immunoglobulin nomenclature have been published by various Committees on Nomenclature for Human Immunoglobulins. *Bull. Wld Hlth Org.*, (1964) **30**, 447; (1965) **33**, 721; (1966) **35**, 953; (1968) **38**, 151; (1969) **41**, 975.

2 STRUCTURE OF IMMUNOGLOBULINS

2.1 Introduction and General Considerations

Although myeloma proteins have made a major contribution to our knowledge of immunoglobulin structure, it was work on pooled rabbit IgG which provided the basis for many present-day concepts. In 1959, Porter showed that rabbit IgG antibodies could be split by the plant protease papain into three large fragments and, furthermore, that these fragments could be separated by ion-exchange chromatography. Two of these fragments were identical and retained univalent antigen-binding capacity (now known as Fab—Fragment antigen binding), whereas the third fragment could be crystallized (now called Fc—Fragment crystalline). The latter fragment has been shown subsequently to be associated with various effector or adjunctive functions of the antibody molecule. Examples of such functions are the binding of the complement protein C1q, macrophage binding, and membrane transmission. The effector functions of immunoglobulins are discussed in detail in Section 3 of this chapter.

Chemical methods of separating the constituent peptide chains of immunoglobulins were described by Edelman and Poulik (1961), and by Fleischman et

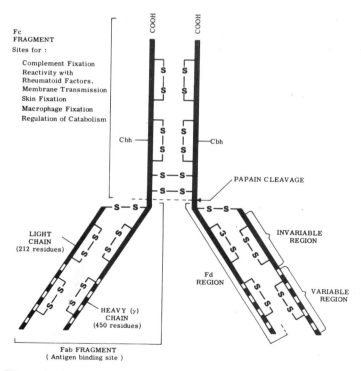

Figure 1 Schematic representation of the four-chain structure of human IgG1 showing inter and intra-chain disulphide bridges, papain fragments, and location of effector functions

al. (1961) and shortly afterwards Porter (1962) proposed a four-chain model for immunoglobulin molecules based on two distinct types of polypeptide chain. This basic four-chain model, which is illustrated in Figure 1, appears to occur throughout the vertebrate kingdom and comprises two small (light) polypeptide chains (molecular weight 22 000) and two larger (heavy) polypeptide chains (molecular weight 50 000–77 000). The heavy chains are invariably covalently bound through disulphide bridges, and usually each heavy chain is bound similarly to a light chain. Occasionally, however, the disulphide bridges between heavy and light chains are absent, and instead the light chains are linked covalently. This is the case with certain IgA molecules in man and the mouse. In all cases, noncovalent forces also help to maintain overall molecular stability.

The light chains are common to all classes of immunoglobulin whereas the heavy chains have the antigenic, immunological, and chemical characteristics of only one of the five classes. The heavy chains characteristic of immunoglobulin chains are designated by appropriate Greek letters—γ chains for IgG, α for IgA, μ for IgM, δ for IgD, and ε for IgE. The light chains of most vertebrates have been shown to exist in two antigenically distinct forms called Kappa (κ type) and lambda (λ type). In any one molecule, both light chains are of the same type and hybrid molecules have never been observed. Both types are present usually in any one individual but the $\kappa : \lambda$ ratio differs from species to species, from class to class, and from subclass to subclass. Thus for human immunoglobulins, the overall ratio is 6:4 but for circulating human IgD it is 2:8. The ratio of light chain types in each of the four subclasses of human IgG is shown in Table 2. In the serum of other animals, the proportions of κ and λ chains range from more than 95 per cent λ chains in the horse to more than 95 per cent κ chains in the mouse. There is evidence that the relative proportions of κ and λ chains change during immunization. This is presumably a reflection of the particular classes and subclasses involved at different stages of the immune response.

Table 2 κ and λ-light chains in human IgG subclasses

Human subclass	$\kappa : \lambda$ ratio	
	a	b
IgG1	2·41	1·42
IgG2	1·10	0·96
IgG3	1·12	1·25
IgG4	5·0	7·0

a data from Terry *et al.* (1965)
b data from Schur (1972)

The realization that serum myeloma proteins and urinary Bence–Jones proteins represent pathological counterparts of normal intact immunoglobulins and free light chains, respectively (Edelman and Gally, 1962), initiated the application of protein-sequencing techniques to these proteins, and many sequences for several species are now available. Only selected sequences are

5

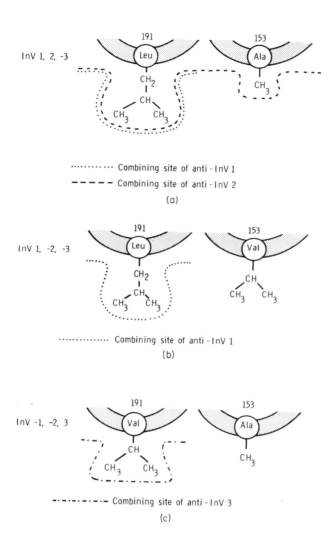

················ Combining site of anti - InV 1
− − − − − Combining site of anti - InV 2

(a)

················ Combining site of anti - InV 1

(b)

− ·· − ·· − Combining site of anti - InV 3

(c)

Figure 2 InV (or Km) antigens and amino acid sequence. Antisera that detect the InV1 (Km (1)) antigen probably interact with a leucine residue at position 191, but do not encompass residue 153. In contrast, antisera to InV2 (Km (2)) recognize the leucine residue at position 191, but also encompass an alanine residue at position 153 (a). If the alanine residue is replaced by valine the anti-InV2 (Km (2)) reagent is no longer able to recognize the complete antigenic determinant, possibly because of steric hindrance by the larger valine residue (b). The third InV allotype (InV3 or Km (3)) is expressed when a valine residue occurs at position 191 and appears to be independent of residue 153, although this is uncertain (c)

6

included in this review but the interested reader can obtain information from the annually updated *Atlas of Protein Structure* (Dayhoff, M. O., ed.), National Biomedical Research Foundation, Silver Spring, Maryland, U.S.A.

The work of Hilschmann and Craig (1965), Baglioni *et al.* (1966), Milstein (1966), and Putnam *et al.* (1966) established the important principle that when light chains of the same type (and from the same species) are sequenced they are seen to comprise two distinct regions. The C-terminal half of the chain (approximately 107 amino acid residues) does not vary except for certain minor differences which reflect either allotypic or isotypic variations. In human κ-chains, for example, alternative amino acid residues may occur at positions 191 and 153 of the peptide chain. These alternative residues correlate with the allotypic antigens InV1, InV2, and InV3 (now called Km (1), Km (2), and Km (3)) as illustrated schematically in Figure 2.

In the case of human λ chains, amino acid differences have been noted at positions 190 and 152, and these correlate with the so-called Oz and Kern

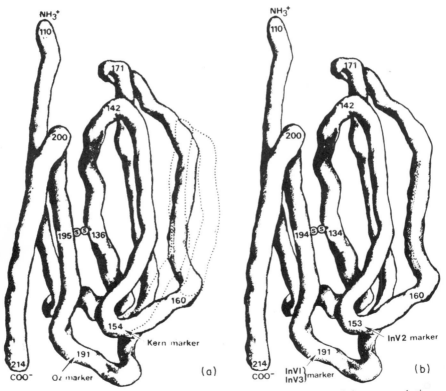

Figure 3 Model of C-terminal half of a human λ light chain (*a*) and, by extrapolation, a similar model for human κ light chain (*b*) showing the basic 'immunoglobulin fold' in both. The approximate location of residues which determine Oz and Kern isotypes and the InV (or Km) allotypes are indicated. The dotted line indicates the position of the extra loop in the V_L region. Modified, with permission, from Poljak (1975)

markers. Unlike the InV (or Km) markers, however, these are both isotypic antigens, that is, all normal individuals have both Oz(+) and Oz(−), and Kern(+) and Kern(−) λ chains.

Recent X-ray crystallographic analyses indicate that each of these amino acid residues is located at the surface and available to the external environment (see Figure 3, and Chapter 7).

In contrast to the C-terminal half of the light polypetide chain the N-terminal region shows much sequence variability. However, the variability observed is not distributed evenly throughout the length of the region. Some positions in the sequence show exceptional variability, and in both κ and λ light chains such hypervariable regions are located near positions 30, 50, 95, and 106 (see Figure 4). It is now generally accepted that such hypervariable residues are involved directly in the formation of the antigen binding site. A feature associated with hypervariable regions is the presence of adjacent constant residues, particularly cysteine, glycine, and tryptophan. These residues are sometimes called 'framework' residues and are thought to create the necessary rigid framework near which apparently unrestricted amino acid variability can occur.

In addition to the hypervariable residues, the N-terminal half of light chains is composed of residues showing a more restricted variation in different proteins. Indeed when sequences are examined for evidence of homology, it is found that the variable regions of both κ and λ chains are divisible into subgroups. In man, κ

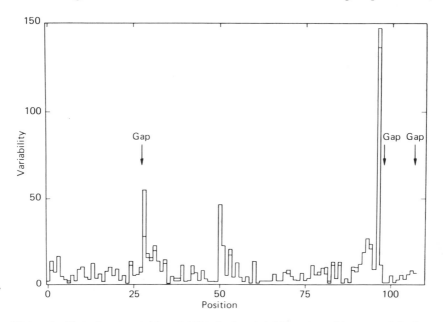

Figure 4 Plot of amino acid variability in the variable region of immunoglobulin light chains according to sequence number. Extra amino acids occur in some sequences and to enhance the comparison these have been excluded as indicated by the arrows. Reproduced from Wu and Kabat (1970), with permission

Table 3 Prototype N-terminal sequences of the subgroups of human κ and λ-light chains

Subgroups	Sequence
κ chains	
$V_\kappa I$	Asp-Ile -Gln-Met-Thr-Gln-Ser-Pro-Ser-Ser-Leu-Ser-Ala-Ser-Val-Gly-Asp- Arg-Val-Thr
$V_\kappa II$	Glu-Ile -Val-Leu-Thr-Gln-Ser-Pro-Gly-Thr-Leu-Ser-Leu-Ser-Pro-Gly-Glu- Arg-Ala-Thr
$V_\kappa III$	Asp-Ile -Val-Met-Thr-Gln-Ser-Pro-Leu-Ser-Leu-Pro-Val-Thr-Pro-Gly-Glu- Pro-Ala-Ser
λ chains	
$V_\lambda I$	*Glp-Ser-Val-Leu-Thr-Gln-Pro-Pro-( )-Ser-Val-Ser-Gly-Ala-Pro-Gly-Gln- Arg-Val-Thr
$V_\lambda II$	*Glp-Ser-Ala-Leu-Thr-Gln-Pro-Ala-( )-Ser-Val-Ser-Gly-Ser-Pro-Gly-Gln- Ser-Ile -Thr
$V_\lambda III$	( )-Tyr-Val-Leu-Thr-Gln-Pro-Pro-( )-Ser-Val-Ser-Val-Ser-Pro-Gly-Gln- Thr-Ala-Ser
$V_\lambda IV$	*Glp-Ser-Ala-Leu-Thr-Gln-Pro-Pro-( )-Ser-Ala-Ser-Gly-Ser-Pro-Gly-Gln- Ser-Val-Thr
$V_\lambda V$	( )-Ser-Glu-Leu-Thr-Gln-Pro-Pro-( )-Ala-Val-Ser-Val-Ala-Leu-Gly-Gln- Thr-Val-Arg

* Residue derived from pyrrolid-2-one-5-carboxylic acid

chains fall into three subgroups and λ chains into five. Prototype sequences of the first 20 residues of such subgroups are illustrated in Table 3.

Sequence studies on heavy chains of monoclonal human immunoglobulins have revealed that, in common with the light chains, there is a V region at the N-terminus of the peptide chain. Generally, V_H regions are slightly longer than V_L regions, comprising 118–124 amino acid residues and having four regions of hypervariability between residues 31–37, 51–68, 84–91, and 101–110. A point of major interest is that V_H-region sequences seem to be shared by all classes. Three V_H subgroups ($V_H I$, $V_H II$, and $V_H III$), have been recognized and within a subgroup sequence homology is of the order of 80–95 per cent (hypervariable regions excluded). The concentration of the heavy chains of the $V_H III$ subgroup in normal immunoglobulin (20 per cent of all heavy chains) is close to the frequency of myeloma proteins of the $V_H III$ subgroup. However, a high proportion of IgA proteins studied (75 per cent) seem to belong to the $V_H III$ subgroup, suggesting that the association between a V-region subgroup and the class-specific C region is not entirely random.

A suggestion by Dreyer and Bennett (1965), that two genes control the synthesis of each immunoglobulin chain is now generally accepted, although genetically unorthodox. According to this view, one gene codes for the constant part of the chain and another for the variable portion. The genes are then brought together by an unknown mechanism and, thereafter, function as a single unit. Studies in several species suggest that there are three distinct linkage groups of immunoglobulin structural genes. These determine the primary structure of κ, λ, and heavy chains (see Figure 5). Within any linkage group any V-region subgroup gene can associate with any C-region gene (Kohler *et al.*, 1970), although some associations may be preferred (for example, IgA–V_HIII).

Recently, it has been suggested that three, rather than two, structural genes may interact to produce each immunoglobulin peptide chain (Capra and Kindt, 1975). According to this hypothesis a limited number of *group one* genes would code for the relatively invariant portions of the V region (perhaps one for each subgroup), a larger number of *group two* genes would encode hypervariable regions, and a small number of *group three* genes would code for the C regions. This hypothesis is elaborated in more detail by one of the authors elsewhere in this volume (see Sogn and Kindt, Chapter 4).

As shown in Figure 1 there are two intra-chain disulphide bridges in the light chain—one in the variable and one in the constant region. Similarly, there are four such bridges in the heavy (γ) chain, which is twice the length of a light chain. Each bridge encloses a peptide loop of 60–70 amino acid residues and if the amino

[margin annotation: isulfide ridge]

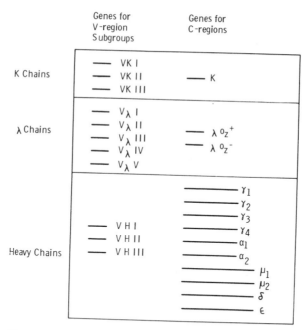

Figure 5 Minimum number of genetic systems for human immunoglobulin synthesis. Each box encloses a set of genes (represented by bars) which are probably linked. One V-region gene and one C-region gene contribute to each immunoglobulin chain, and other genes (not shown) may contribute to hypervariability. The heavy, κ, and λ-chain systems appear to be three unlinked systems. In the figure, genes are labelled by the name of their protein product

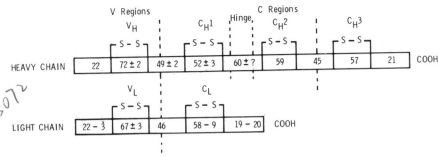

Figure 6 Schematic diagram of human IgG homology regions showing number of amino acid residues enclosed by each disulphide bridge (range for four subclasses shown). Modified from Milstein and Svasti (1971)

acid sequences of these loops are compared within a given heavy chain a striking degree of homology is revealed. Each loop represents the central portion of a so-called homology region or 'domain' which comprises some 110 amino acid residues. In the light chain, these regions are called V_L and C_L, respectively, for the variable and constant regions. In the heavy chain, the N-terminal homology region is called the V_H region and there are at least three homology regions in the constant part of the chain called C_H1, C_H2, and C_H3 (see Figure 6). There are known to be three constant homology regions in γ and α heavy chains and four such regions in μ and ε chains. There are probably four in δ chains also. A specific nomenclature may be used to describe the homology regions of different classes, for example $C_\gamma1$, $C_\gamma2$, and $C_\gamma3$ for IgG, and $C_\mu1$, $C_\mu2$, $C_\mu3$, and $C_\mu4$ for IgM. The variation in size of the homology regions of human IgG subclasses is indicated in Figure 6. This shows that the V_H and V_L disulphide-bridged loops are larger than the C-region loops of these chains. Furthermore the regions between loops are of comparable size except that between the C_H1 and C_H2 loops which is longer (especially in IgG3). The latter feature (sometimes called the 'hinge' region) is common to the four-domain IgG and IgA molecules, but is not shared apparently with the five-domain IgM and IgE molecules. In IgG and IgA, the hinge region shows no sequence homology with any other part of the polypeptide structure and appears to have evolved independently. An intriguing possibility proposed recently by Bennich (personal communication) is that the hinge regions of IgG and IgA represent 'collapsed' domains, thus these regions are the equivalent of $C_\varepsilon2$ and $C_\mu2$ domains.

Edelman and Gall (1969) proposed that each homology region is folded into a compact globular structure and linked to neighbouring domains by more loosely folded portions of peptide chain. Furthermore, it was suggested by Edelman (1970) that each homology region has evolved to fulfil a specific function, for example, antigen binding would be the major function of the V_L and V_H domains. There is much evidence to support this concept. This will be discussed in Section 3.

In the last five years, the three-dimensional structure of immunoglobulins has been under active investigation and high resolution data are now available for the

Fab regions of human IgG1 (Amzel *et al.*, 1974) and mouse IgA (Segal *et al.*, 1974), as well as human λ Bence–Jones dimer (Edmundson *et al.*, 1974). Much of this work is reviewed elsewhere in this volume (Richards *et al.*, Chapter 2), but the major conclusions of this work are summarized here.

Within each homology region two roughly parallel β-pleated sheets surround a tightly coiled internal structure of hydrophobic side chains. The two β sheets are linked covalently by the intra-chain disulphide bridge, and there appears not to be any α-helical structure present. Many of the 'framework' residues of the two variable regions (V_H and V_L) occur at hairpin bends, or contribute to the intra- and inter-subunit bonds thereby enhancing the overall structural stability. At such positions, only specific amino acids are compatible with the requirements for a constant three-dimensional structure for all homology subunits. On the other hand, the hypervariable portions of the V_L and V_H regions come together at the N-terminal surface of the molecule and appear not to be subject to structural constraints. These combined hypervariable regions are thought to constitute the 'contact residues' of the antigen binding site (see also Feinstein and Beale Chapter 8).

Subclasses of human IgG and IgA exist and probably also of IgM and IgD. Most mammals, with the exception of the rabbit, appear to have two or more subclasses of IgG but there are no clear relationships between species suggesting that the subclasses are relatively recent evolutionary events which have arisen independently in each species. All healthy individuals have the subclass variants of IgG and IgA in their serum and the antigenic markers of these proteins are termed isotypic markers. Certain genetic markers are also identifiable. These are inherited as autosomal codominant factors called allotypic markers and are found on γ chains (Gm antigens), α chains (Am antigens) and κ light chains (Km antigens).

Table 4 Physicochemical properties of human immunoglobulins

Immuno-globulin	Heavy chain	Sedimen-tation constant (S)	Total molecular weight	Molecular weight of heavy chain	Number of heavy chain domains	Carbo-hydrate (per cent)
IgG1	γ_1	7	146 000	51 000	4	2–3
IgG2	γ_2	7	146 000	51 000	4	2–3
IgG3	γ_3	7	170 000	60 000	4*	2–3
IgG4	γ_4	7	146 000	51 000	4	2–3
IgM	μ	19	970 000	65 000	5	12
IgA1	α_1	7	160 000	56 000	4	7–11
IgA2	α_2	7	160 000	52 000	4	7–11
sIgA†	α_1 or α_2	11	385 000	52 000–56 000	4	7–11
IgD	δ	7	184 000	69 700	5	9–14
IgE	ε	8	188 000	72 500	5	12

* The hinge region of IgG3 may incorporate an intra-chain disulphide bridge but this would not constitute a domain of 110 residues
† secretory IgA

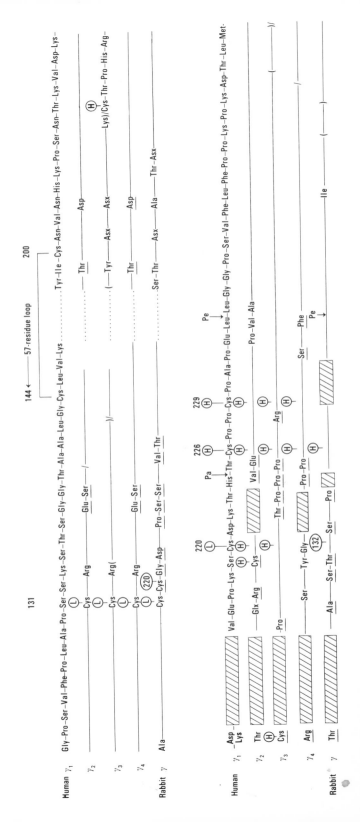

Figure 7 Partial sequences of the three C_H regions of four subclasses of human γ chains and the rabbit γ chain. The symbols L or H adjacent to a Cys residue indicate a disulphide bond linking that Cys to a light or heavy chain, respectively. Other Cys residues form intra-chain disulphide bridges. Carbohydrate (CBH) is attached to an asparagine residue (no. 297). Residue numbering according to the Eu sequence of Edelman *et al.* (1969). Pa and Pe indicate cleavage points of papain and pepsin, respectively. Allotype related substitutions are indicated by alternative residues. Within the 57 residue C_H1 loop there is data for γ₁ and rabbit γ only, and this section has been omitted. Closed boxes indicate gaps introduced to maximize homology. Solid lines indicate identical residues. Data modified from Nisonoff *et al.* (1975) with additional material from Wolfenstein-Todel *et al.* (1976)

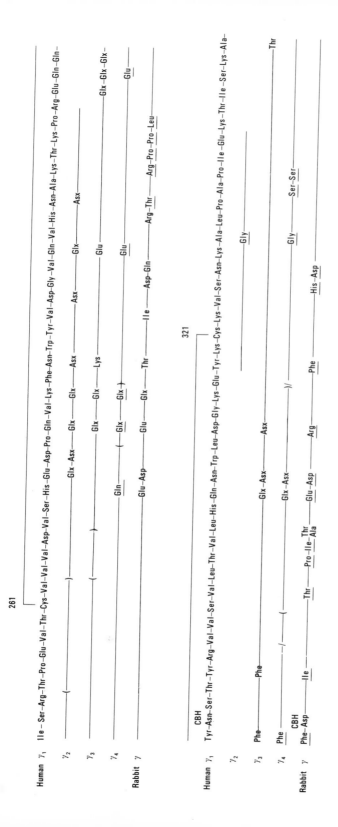

367

Human γ₁: Lys-Gly-Gln-Pro-Arg-Glu-Pro-Gln-Val-Tyr-Thr-Leu-Pro-Pro-Ser-Arg-Asp-Leu-Thr-Lys-Asn-Gln-Val-Ser-Leu-Thr-Cys-Leu-Val-Lys-Gly-Phe-Tyr-Pro-Ser-Asp-Ile-Ala-Val-Glu-Trp-Glu-Ser-Asn-

(above: Asp—Glu / Met / Glu)

γ₂: — Asx—Glx — — Asx-

γ₃: — Glx — Glx — — Glx — (Asx)

γ₄: — Gln —

Rabbit γ: Arg —Glu— Leu —Lys— Met-Gly — Pro-Gln — Gln-Leu-Ser-Ser-Arg-Ser — Ser — Gly — Lys-Asp

425

Human γ₁: Asp-Gly-Glu-Pro-Glu-Asn-Tyr-Lys-Thr-Thr-Pro-Pro-Val-Leu-Asp-Ser-Asp-Gly-Ser-Phe-Phe-Leu-Tyr-Ser-Lys-Leu-Thr-Val-Asp-Lys-Ser-Arg-Trp-Gln-Glu-Gly-Asn-Val-Phe-Ser-Cys-Ser-Val-Met-

γ₂:

γ₃: Asx — Glx-Asx — Met — Asx — Asx — Glx-Glx — Asx-Ile

γ₄: Asx — Glx — Glx-Asx) — Arg — (Glx-Glx — Asx —)

Rabbit γ: Gly-Lys-Ala-Glu-Asp-Asp — Ala — Trp — Arg — Ser — Pro-Thr — Glu — Arg — Asp — Thr

446 ●

Human γ₁: His-Glu-Ala-Leu-His-Asn-His-Tyr-Thr-Gln-Lys-Ser-Leu-Ser-Leu-Ser-Pro-Gly(COOH)

γ₂:

γ₃: Arg-Phe — Leu

γ₄: Leu

Rabbit γ: Ile — Arg

The major physicochemical properties of the classes and subclasses of human immunoglobulin are shown in Table 4. The structural characteristics of each class will now be considered in greater detail.

2.2 Structure of Immunoglobulin G

2.2.1 Human Immunoglobulin G

IgG is the major immunoglobulin in normal human serum accounting for 70–75 per cent of the total immunoglobulin pool. Isolated pooled IgG is a monomeric protein with a sedimentation coefficient (s_{20°, w) of 6·6 S and a molecular weight of 146 000. However, studies of subclass proteins have indicated that IgG3 proteins are slightly larger than the other subclasses (see Table 4). Following electrophoresis IgG shows a broad range of mobilities from slow γ to α_2. This range of net charge (partly a reflection of the subclass content) is also seen on isoelectric focusing and ion-exchange chromatography.

Four subclasses of human IgG (IgG1, IgG2, IgG3, and IgG4) have been recognized and occur in the approximate proportions of 66, 23, 7, and 4 per cent, respectively. These subclasses cross-react antigenically but also possess subclass-specific antigenic determinants in the C_H regions. These antigenic differences are, of course, reflected in the amino acid sequences of heavy chains from myeloma proteins of different subclasses. The first human γ chain to be sequenced completely was the γ_1 chain of the Eu protein (Edelman *et al.*, 1969), and the numbering system for this chain is used frequently as a basis for comparisons between γ-chain sequences. Partial C-region sequences of human γ_1, γ_2, γ_3, and γ_4 chains and rabbit γ chain are shown in Figure 7. Inspection of these sequences shows that each protein has three homology regions or domains. Each of these domains encompasses a disulphide-bridged loop of 52–59 residues (see Figure 6). More variable than the number of residues within the loops is the number *between* the loops. For example in IgG1, IgG2, and IgG4 there are 10–15 more residues between the C_H1 and C_H2 disulphide loops than between the C_H2 and C_H3 loops. These extra residues occur in what has become known as the hinge or bridge region, and it is here that structural and sequential differences between subclasses are greatest. Two amino acid residues are especially frequent in this region, namely half-cystine and proline. Although in IgG1 the half-cystine at residue 220 contributes to the light–heavy chain bridge, most of the half-cystine residues in the hinge region are those involved in inter-heavy chain disulphide bridges. There are two inter-chain disulphide bonds between both γ_1 and γ_4 chains, and four between γ_2 chains. The number of such bonds in IgG3 is still controversial; estimates range from five (Frangione and Milstein, 1968) to 15 (Michaelsen, 1973). It is possible that the hinge-region peptide of IgG3 originally sequenced by Frangione and Milstein (1968), and containing five half-cystines, is triplicated to give the 15 half-cystines suggested subsequently. This is consistent with the presence of approximately 95 extra amino acid residues in the γ_3 chain and would account for its higher molecular weight of 60 000 (see Table 4). The disulphide-bridge patterns of the human IgG subclasses are illustrated in Figure 8.

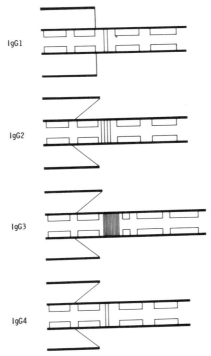

IgG1

IgG2

IgG3

IgG4

Figure 8 Gross structure of human IgG subclasses showing heavy and light polypeptide chains (long and short thick lines) and both inter and intra-chain disulphide bridges (thin lines). The positions of the bridges are based on comparisons with homologous sequences in human IgG1 molecules. Data for IgG3 are tentative

The hinge regions of the γ chains are also rich in proline (see Figure 7), and it has been suggested by Welscher (1970) that this amino acid stabilizes the structure of the hinge. Whether or not this is the case, there is evidence that the peptide structure is exposed and particularly susceptible to proteolysis in this region. A wide range of proteolytic enzymes cleave IgG molecules in the hinge region but the most extensively used enzymes have been papain and pepsin. Using papain, Fc and Fab fragments can be obtained from all four IgG subclasses, although there are marked differences in susceptibility to the enzyme; IgG3 is the most susceptible followed by IgG1, IgG4, and IgG2. The enzyme cleaves the γ chains of each subclass on the N-terminal side of the inter-heavy chain disulphide bonds but can also cleave at other points. For example, a fragment derived from the C_H3 domain and called Fc′ is detected frequently after

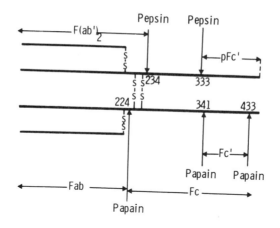

Figure 9 Pepsin and papain cleavage points of human IgG1. Numbers refer to the amino acid on the N-terminal side of the bond cleaved and are based on the Eu sequence of Edelman *et al.* (1969). Reproduced, with permission, from Stanworth and Turner (1973)

prolonged papain digestion (Turner and Bennich, 1968). The major papain cleavage points of human IgG1 are illustrated in Figure 9.

Pepsin at pH 4·0–4·5 can cleave γ chains also in the hinge region, but in this case the susceptible bond is on the C-terminal side of the inter-heavy chain disulphide bridges (see Figure 9 for cleavage point of IgG1). This yields a divalent fragment called F(ab′)₂ which essentially consists of the two Fab regions held together by the hinge region. At pH 4·0, the rest of the Fc region is destroyed, but at pH 4·5 a fragment corresponding closely to the C_H3 domain of each subclass (pFc′) is readily obtained (Turner *et al.*, 1970).

The generation of Fc′ and pFc′ by cleavage of peptide bonds between the C_H2 and C_H3 regions suggests that controlled enzymic cleavage between other domains may permit their isolation for structural and biological studies. Such indeed appears to be the case and methods for isolating the C_H2 domain using brief exposure to trypsin (Yasmeen *et al.*, 1973) or treatment with pepsin at a high temperature (70°, pH 4·5, 50 minutes incubation, enzyme:substrate ratio 1:100) have been reported (Seon and Pressman, 1975).

An apparently large structural difference between human IgG1 and the other IgG subclasses is the location of the heavy chain half-cystine which links to the light chain half-cystine. This is residue 220 in IgG1 but a residue homologous to position 131 in the other subclasses (and indeed in most other immunoglobulin classes). X-Ray crystallographic analysis of the human IgG1 protein (NEW) to a resolution of 0·2 nm (Amzel *et al.*, 1974) has, however, shown that positions 131 and 220 of the γ₁ chain in fact are spatially very close and that the overall three-

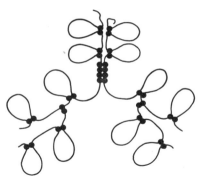

Figure 10 Schematic diagram of human IgG2 showing both intra and inter-chain disulphide bridges between $\frac{1}{2}$-cystine residues (●●). Note the proximity of the C-terminus of the light chain to both the N-terminal and C-terminal sides of the $C_H 1$ loop

dimensional structure of the molecule is not influenced greatly whichever alternative operates. This point is illustrated diagrammatically in Figure 10.

All subclasses of IgG contain carbohydrate and it is probable that this is located on the outside of the $C_H 2$ domain and (by extrapolation from studies on IgG1) attached to an asparagine at residue 297 of each heavy chain (see Figure 7). The obligatory triplet sequence Asn–X–Ser/Thr occurs at positions 297–299 of both γ_1 and γ_4 chains (Edelman *et al.*, 1969; Pink *et al.*, 1970), but not elsewhere in the C regions of these proteins. Although there is a wide variation in the sugar groups associated with IgG myeloma proteins, there is no evidence that this variation is linked in a specific way to the subclasses.

The ease with which papain cleaves the IgG molecule into two Fab fragments and one Fc fragment suggests that the molecule has a natural tripartite structure. This is confirmed apparently by the electron micrographs obtained by Valentine and Green (1967). These workers used a rabbit antibody with specificity for a DNP hapten. When the antibody was mixed with the bivalent hapten DNP-NH-$(CH_2)_n$-NH-DNP (where n was 8 or more), a number of closed structures including cyclic dimers, trimers, tetramers, and pentamers was visualized readily in the electron microscope (see Fearon and Beale, chapter 8). These micrographs suggest that IgG is a Y-shaped molecule in which the three limbs represent the Fc and the two Fab regions. The angle between the Fab limbs in these complexes varies between 10° and 180°. These results confirm earlier work by Feinstein and Rowe (1965) which suggested a highly flexible structure.

A large number of allotypic antigens (Gm markers) has now been described for human γ chains. These are listed in Table 5 together with the subclass to which the antigen is restricted. A feature of the Gm system, which has not yet been described in any other animal allotype system, is the association of so-called 'iso-allotypes' with many Gm antigens. Such antigens are shared by two or more

Table 5 Established Gm allotypes of human immunoglobulin G

Original nomenclature	New nomenclature	IgG subclass
a	G1m(a)	IgG1
x	G1m(x)	IgG1
f	G1m(f)	IgG1
z	G1m(z)	IgG1
n	G2m(n)	IgG2
g	G3m(g)	IgG3
b^0	G3m(b^0)	IgG3
b^1	G3m(b^1)	IgG3
b^3	G3m(b^3)	IgG3
b^4	G3m(b^4)	IgG3
b^5	G3m(b^5)	IgG3
c^3	G3m(c^3)	IgG3
c^5	G3m(c^5)	IgG3
s	G3m(s)	IgG3
t	G3m(t)	IgG3

subclasses and are structurally antithetic to a Gm marker in one subclass only. The most widely studied example is nG1m(a), an antigen present on all IgG2 and IgG3 proteins but only on IgG1 molecules lacking the Gm(a) antigen. A plausible explanation for the existence of both classical allotypic antigens and antithetic antigens is that Gm antigens have arisen following a mutation in a portion of the C-region gene controlling a subclass-specific segment of the γ polypeptide chain. G1m(z) and G1m(f) at residue number 214 of the γ_1 chain are examples of such classical allelic antigens. In contrast, mutations in a part of the gene controlling

Table 6 Probable structural location of some human γ-chain allotypes and iso-allotypes

Allotype or Iso-allotype	Chain	Homology region	Sequence	Amino acid
G1m(a)	γ_1	$C_\gamma 3$	355–358	Arg-*Asp*-Glu-*Leu*
nG1m(a)	$\gamma_1, \gamma_2, \gamma_3$	$C_\gamma 3$	355–358	Arg-Glu-Glu-Met
G1m(f)	γ_1	$C_\gamma 1$	214	Arg
G1m(z)	γ_1	$C_\gamma 1$	214	Lys
nG4m(a)	$\gamma_1, \gamma_3, \gamma_4$	$C_\gamma 2$	309	Val-Leu-His
nG4m(b)	γ_2, γ_4	$C_\gamma 2$	309	Val-His
G3m(g)	γ_3	$C_\gamma 2$	296*	Tyr
nG3m(g)	γ_2, γ_3	$C_\gamma 2$	296*	Phe
G3m(b^0)	γ_3	$C_\gamma 3$	436**	Phe
nG3m(b^0)	$\gamma_1, \gamma_2, \gamma_3$	$C_\gamma 3$	436**	Tyr

* and ** Correlative sequence differences observed in incompletely sequenced chains.

regions common to other subclasses may give rise to a genetic marker in one subclass—for example G1m(a)—but the antithetic marker (nG1m(a)) is shared with two other subclasses (IgG2 and IgG3).

A combination of peptide mapping, mild proteolytic fragmentation, and amino acid analysis has permitted the partial structural localization of several Gm and antithetic antigens. Some of these data are summarized in Table 6. Extrapolation of the X-ray crystallographic data on the constant (C_H1) homology region of Fab fragments suggests that if a similar folding of the γ-polypeptide chain exists in the C_H2 and C_H3 regions then all of the antigens listed in Table 6 will occupy surface positions, usually near bends and corners (see also Fearon and Beale, Chapter 8).

The structural localization of effector sites in the IgG molecule is still in its infancy but there has been limited progress in the case of both the complement-fixing site and the macrophage/monocyte-binding site. These data are considered in more detail in Section 3.

2.2.2 Immunoglobulin G from Other Species

The IgG class of several mammalian species has now been studied in some detail. This section will deal briefly with some of the points of major interest; readers requiring a more detailed review are recommended to consult Nisonoff *et al.* (1975).

The known subclasses and overall structure of IgG from rabbit, mouse, guinea-pig, and goat are shown in Figure 11. The rabbit is unusual in that its IgG exists as a single major subclass. The protein has a single inter-heavy chain disulphide bond, two intra-chain disulphide loops in the C_1 region and a light–heavy bond which joins the heavy chain near the V–C junction. Much of the early elucidation of immunoglobulin structure was performed on rabbit IgG (see Porter, 1959; Hill *et al.*, 1966).

Four subclasses of IgG have been described in the mouse (IgG1, IgG2a, IgG2b, and IgG3). The availability of myeloma proteins representative of each of these subclasses has permitted extensive structural work to be carried out. IgG2a (quantitatively the most important) and IgG2b are structurally similar and are difficult to isolate from each other. Mouse IgG3 is present at low concentrations and is the least studied of the four subclasses. All four subclasses are cleaved readily by papain to give Fc and Fab fragments.

Two major subclasses of guinea-pig IgG (called IgG1 and IgG2) have been described, and a third minor subclass is suggested by the work of Parish (1970). IgG1 and IgG2 of guinea-pig differ extensively in the structure of the Fc regions and also in their biological effector functions. Both subclasses may be digested readily with papain to give Fc and Fab fragments.

Studies on the inter-chain disulphide bridges of goat IgG (Strausbauch *et al.*, 1971) show that it is similar to rabbit IgG with a single bond between the heavy chains and light–heavy bonds to residue 131 of the heavy chains (see Figure 11).

Recent work from the laboratory of Marchalonis (Atwell and Marchalonis,

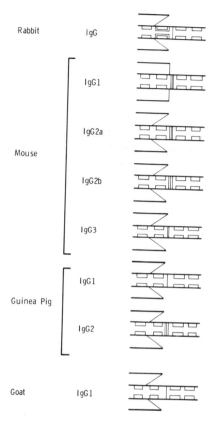

Rabbit   IgG

Mouse   IgG1

IgG2a

IgG2b

IgG3

Guinea Pig   IgG1

IgG2

Goat   IgG1

Figure 11 Gross structure of IgG subclasses from rabbit, mouse, guinea pig, and goat. Heavy and light polypeptide chains are indicated by the long and short thick lines, respectively, and inter and intra-chain disulphide bridges by thin lines. Data from De Préval *et al.* (1970); O'Donnell *et al.* (1970); Grey *et al.* (1971); Oliveira and Lamm (1971); Svasti and Milstein (1972)

1975, 1976) suggests that the low molecular weight non-IgM antibodies of lower vertebrates, including amphibians, reptiles, and birds, are distinct from the IgG class of mammals. The protein present in the serum of lower vertebrates has light chains which are of normal molecular weight (23 000) but the heavy chains are larger than the mammalian ones with a molecular weight of 61 400 in the case of the marine toad *Bufo marinus*. This gives a total molecular weight of 168 000 for the intact four-chain molecule which is close to that of the human IgG3. It is possible that the human subclass has a close phylogenetic relationship with the low

					100										110									120								
κ		Ser	Thr	Leu	Thr	Leu	Ser	—	Lys	Ala	—	Asp	Tyr	—	Glu	Lys	His	Lys	Val	Tyr	Ala	—	Cys	Glu	Val	Thr	His	Gln	Gly	—	Leu	Ser	Ser
λ		Ser	Tyr	Leu	Ser	Leu	Thr	Pro	—	—	Glu	Gln	Trp	Lys	Ser	—	His	Arg	Ser	Tyr	Ser	—	Cys	Gln	Val	Thr	His	Glu	Gly	—	—	Ser	Thr
γ_1	C1	Ser	Val	Val	Thr	Val	Pro	Ser	—	Ser	—	—	Ser	Leu	—	Gly	Thr	Gln	Thr	Tyr	Ile	—	Cys	Asn	Val	Asn	His	Lys	Pro	—	Ser	Asn	Thr
	C2	Ser	Val	Leu	Thr	Val	Leu	—	—	His	Gln	Asp	Trp	Leu	Asp	Gly	—	Lys	Glu	Tyr	Lys	—	Cys	Lys	Val	Ser	Asn	Lys	Ala	—	Leu	Pro	Ala
	C3	Ser	Lys	Leu	Thr	Val	Asp	—	Lys	Ser	—	Arg	Trp	Gln	Gln	Gly	—	Asn	Val	Phe	Ser	—	Cys	Ser	Val	Met	His	Glu	Ala	—	Leu	His	Asn
μ	C1	Ser	Gln	Val	Leu	Leu	Pro	Ser	Lys	—	—	Asp	Val	Met	Gln	Gly	Thr	Asn	Glu	His	Val	Val	Cys	Lys	Val	Glx	His	Pro	—	—	Asx	Gly	Asx
	C2	Ser	Thr	Leu	Thr	Ile	Lys	Glu	—	Ser	—	Asx	Trp	Leu	Ser	Gln	—	Ser	Met	Phe	Thr	—	Cys	Arg	Val	Asp	His	Arg	Gly	—	Leu	—	Thr
	C3	—	—	—	—	—	—	—	—	Glu	Asx	Asx	Trp	Asn	Ser	Gly	—	Glu	Arg	Phe	Thr	—	Cys	Thr	Val	Thr	His	Thr	Asp	—	Leu	Pro	Ser
	C4	Ser	Ile	Leu	Thr	Val	Ser	—	—	Glu	Glu	Glu	Trp	Asn	Thr	Gly	—	Glu	Thr	Tyr	Thr	—	Cys	Val	Val	Ala	His	Glu	Ala	—	Leu	Pro	Asn
α_1	C1	Ser	Gln	Leu	Thr	Leu	Pro	—	—	Ala	Thr	Glx	[Cys]	Leu	Ala	Gly	—	Lys	Ser	Val	Thr	—	Cys	His	Val	Lys	His	Tyr	Thr	—	Asx	Pro	Ser
	C2	Ser	Val	Leu	Ser	Gly	[Cys]	—	—	Ala	Gln	Pro	Trp	Asp	His	Gly	—	Lys	Thr	Phe	Thr	—	Cys	Thr	Ala	Ala	Tyr	Pro	Glu	—	Ser	Lys	Thr
	C3	Ser	Ile	Leu	Arg	Val	Ala	—	—	Ala	Glx	Asx	Trp	Lys	Lys	Gly	—	Asp	Thr	Phe	Ser	—	Cys	Met	Val	Gly	His	Glu	Ala	—	Leu	Pro	Leu
ε	C1	Ser	Leu	Leu	Thr	Val	Ser	Gly	—	Ala	—	—	Trp	Ala	Lys	—	—	Gln	Met	Phe	Thr	—	Cys	Arg	Val	Ala	His	Thr	Pro	—	Ser	Ser	Thr
	C2	Ser	Glu	Leu	Thr	Leu	Ser	Gln	Lys	His	—	—	Trp	Leu	Ser	Asp	—	Arg	Thr	Tyr	Thr	—	Cys	Glu	Val	Thr	Tyr	Glx	Gly	—	—	His	Thr
	C3	Ser	Thr	Leu	Pro	Val	Gly	Thr	Arg	—	—	Asx	Trp	Ile	Glu	Gly	—	Glu	Thr	Tyr	Glx	—	Cys	Arg	Val	Thr	His	Pro	His	—	Leu	Pro	Arg
	C4	Ser	Arg	Leu	Glu	Val	—	Thr	Arg	Ala	Glu	—	Trp	Gln	Glu	Lys	—	Asp	Glu	Phe	Ile	—	Cys	Arg	Ala	Val	His	Glu	Ala	Ala	Ser	Pro	Ser

			130										140										150									159
κ		Pro	Val	Thr	—	Lys	Ser	Phe	Asn	Arg	Gly	Glu	[Cys]	—																		
λ		—	Val	—	Glu	Lys	Thr	Val	Ala	Pro	Thr	Glu	[Cys]	Ser																		
γ_1	C1	Lys	Val	—	Asp	Lys	Lys	Val	Glu	Pro	Lys	Ser	[Cys]	Asp	Lys	Thr	His	Thr	[Cys]	Pro	Pro	[Cys]	Pro	Ala	Pro							
	C2	Pro	Ile	—	Glu	Lys	Thr	Ile	Ser	Lys	Ala	Lys	Gly	—																		
	C3	His	Tyr	Thr	Gln	Lys	Ser	Leu	Ser	Leu	Ser	Pro	Gly	—																		
μ	C1	Lys	—	—	Glu	Lys	Asp	Val	—	Pro	Leu	Pro	—	—																		
	C2	Phe	Gln	—	Gln	Asx	—	—	Ala	Ser	Ser	Met	[Cys]	—																		
	C3	Pro	Leu	Lys	Gln	—	Thr	Ile	Ser	Arg	Pro	Lys	Gly	—																		
	C4	Arg	Val	Thr	Glu	Arg	Thr	Val	Asp	Lys	Ser	Thr	Gly	Lys	Pro	Thr	Leu	Tyr	Asx	Val	Ser	Leu	Val	Met	Ser	Asx	Thr	Ala	Gly	Thr	[Cys]	Tyr
α_1	C1	—	—	—	Glx	Asx	—	Val	Thr	—	Val	Pro	[Cys]	—	Pro	Val	Pro	Ser	Thr	Pro	Pro	Thr	Pro	Ser	Pro							
																		Ser	Thr	Pro	Pro	Thr	Pro	Ser	Pro	—	—	—	—	Ser	[Cys]	[Cys]
	C2	Pro	Leu	Thr	Ala	—	Thr	Leu	Ser	Lys	—	Ser	Gly	—																		
	C3	Ala	Phe	Thr	Gln	Lys	Thr	Ile	Asp	Arg	Leu	Ala	Gly	Lys	Pro	Thr	His	Val	Asx	Val	Ser	Val	Val	Met	Ala	Glu	Val	Asp	Gly	Thr	[Cys]	Tyr
ε	C1	Asx	Asn	—	Val	Lys	Thr	Phe	Ser	Val	—	—	[Cys]	Ser																		
	C2	Phe	—	—	Glx	Asx	Ser	—	Thr	Lys	—	Lys	[Cys]	Ala																		
	C3	Ala	Leu	—	Met	Arg	Ser	Thr	Thr	Lys	Thr	Ser	Gly	—																		
	C4	Gln	Thr	Val	Gln	Arg	Ala	Val	Ser	Val	Asn	Pro	Gly	Lys																		

Figure 12 Primary amino acids sequence of the constant regions of κ, λ, γ_1, μ, α_1, and ε chains. Gaps have been introduced to maximize homology. Adapted, from Kratzin *et al.* (1975). Reproduced by permission of authors and publishers

molecular weight immunoglobulins of lower vertebrates. However, more detailed structural studies, particularly of the hinge region, are required to establish such a possibility.

2.3 Structure of Immunoglobulin A

2.3.1 Serum Immunoglobulin A

IgA was first identified as β_x-globulin by immunoelectrophoresis of human serum (Graber and Williams, 1953), where it accounts for about 15–20 per cent of the total immunoglobulin pool. In man, more than 80 per cent of IgA occurs as 7 S four-chain monomers ($\alpha_2 L_2$) with the remainder as polymers having sedimentation coefficients of 10, 13, and 15 S. In most mammals, the IgA in serum is predominantly 10 S. IgA polymers may be reduced to four-chain monomers by thiol treatment and are stabilized presumably by inter-monomer disulphide bonds. Monomeric IgA has a molecular weight of 160 000, while the isolated α chains have a molecular weight of 52 000–56 000. This is similar to γ chains which also have four domains per chain.

Two subclasses of IgA—IgA1 and IgA2—have been identified in normal human serum using antisera raised in other species (Feinstein and Franklin, 1966; Kunkel and Prendergast, 1966; Vaerman and Heremans, 1966). In serum, IgA1 is the predominant subclass (80–90 per cent), but in seromucous secretions the α_1 and α_2 chains are present in secretory IgA in approximately equal proportions (Grey et al., 1968). The α_1 and α_2 chains have been reported by Montgomery et al. (1969) and by Dorrington and Rockey (1970) to have slightly different molecular weights (52 000 and 56 000, respectively), although it is not known where the additional residues in the α_2 chain are located.

Recently, the primary structure of a monoclonal human IgA1 protein has been determined in Hilschmann's laboratory (Kratzin et al., 1975; Scholz and Hilschmann, 1975). The α_1 chain of this protein comprises 472 amino acid residues with a V region extending from residue 1 to 119. The C region of the α chain consists of three homology regions each showing sequence homology with the C regions of light chains and other immunoglobulin heavy chains (see Figure 12). A feature shared with IgM is the presence of an additional C-terminal octadecapeptide with a penultimate cysteine which is able to bind covalently to the J chain in polymeric molecules. The $C_\alpha 1$ and $C_\alpha 2$ homology regions are each distinguished by the presence of an additional intra-chain disulphide bridge and in each $C_\alpha 2$ homology region there are two cysteine residues of unknown function. It is possible that these are the residues involved in covalent binding to the secretory component but as yet there is no direct evidence for this. A schematic structure for human serum IgA1 based on the work of Kratzin et al. (1975) is shown in Figure 13. It is in the hinge region that the greatest differences between IgA1 and IgA2 molecules are seen, for example, α_2 chains lack 12 amino acid residues and the two galactosamine-rich carbohydrate moieties which are present in the hinge of α_1 chains (Frangione and Wolfenstein-Todel, 1972).

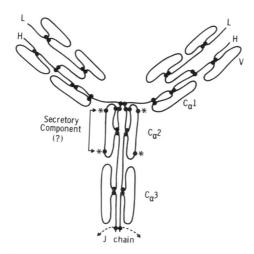

Figure 13 Polypeptide structure of human
IgA1 showing intra and inter-chain disulphide
bridges between $\frac{1}{2}$-cystine residues (●●). The
secretory-component binding role of the cysteine residues in the $C_\alpha 2$ region is speculative

Furthermore, there is a duplicated sequence of seven amino acid residues in the α_1
hinge which does not occur in the α_2 hinge (see Figure 14).

IgA2 molecules exist in two allotypic forms—$A_2m(1)$ and $A_2m(2)$. The $A_2m(1)$
molecules have been shown to possess an unusual molecular structure. The light
chains are disulphide bonded to each other but not to the α chains (Grey *et al.*
1968). There are, however, strong non-covalent forces between the light and
heavy chains. A second Am allotype, which appears to be located in the Fd region
of IgA2 molecules, has been described by Wang *et al.* (1973).

Treatment of IgA with proteolytic enzymes has been relatively unproductive.
Digestion with papain was found by Bernier *et al.* (1965) to yield Fab-like
fragments and, recently, treatment with a streptococcal IgA protease has been
reported to produce both Fab and Fc-like fragments from IgA1 but not from
IgA2 proteins (Plaut *et al.*, 1974).

2.3.2 *Secretory Immunoglobulin A*

In 1963, Chodirker and Tomasi reported that IgA is the predominant
immunoglobulin in seromucous secretions. Such secretory IgA is found only in
external secretions such as saliva, tracheobronchial secretions, colostrum, milk,
and genitourinary secretions. In these secretions, the IgG:IgA ratio is always less
than one, whereas in internal secretions such as synovial, amniotic, pleural, and
cerebrospinal fluids, and in the aqueous humour of the eye the IgA is not of the
secretory type and the IgG:IgA ratio is similar to plasma, that is approximately
5:1.

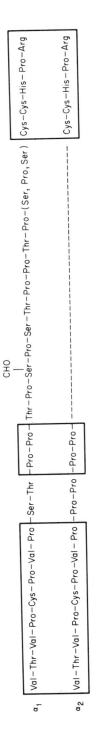

Figure 14 Primary amino acid sequence of human IgA α_1 and α_2 chains in the hinge region of the molecule according to Frangione and Wolfenstein-Todel (1972)

α chain

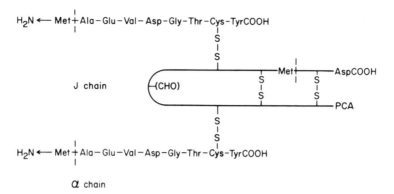

H₂N ⟵ Met┼Ala−Glu−Val−Asp−Gly−Thr−Cys−TyrCOOH

J chain

H₂N ⟵ Met┼Ala−Glu−Val−Asp−Gly−Thr−Cys−TyrCOOH

α chain

Figure 15 Suggested model for attachment of J chain to α chain in
polymeric human IgA. Reproduced from Mestecky *et al.* (1974), with
permission

Secretory IgA exists mainly in the 11 S form and has a molecular weight of
380 000. The complete molecule is made up of two four-chain units of IgA, one
secretory component (molecular weight 70 000) and one J chain (molecular
weight 15 000). It is not at present clear how the various peptide chains are linked

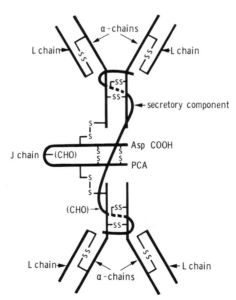

Figure 16 Schematic diagram of human
secretory IgA showing possible arrangement
of IgA monomers, secretory component, and
J chain

together. It is known, however, that the J chain is a product of the plasma cells which synthesize the IgA molecule and that it is added just before secretion. It is also known that the J chain is attached to the penultimate half-cystine of the α chain (Figure 15) and that one or two half-cystines join the J chain to an α chain (Mestecky et al., 1974). As in the case of polymeric IgM (see p. 29), it is not yet clear whether the J chain is linked to two four-chain units of IgA or to one or both heavy chains of a single IgA subunit.

In contrast to the J chain, the secretory component is not synthesized by plasma cells but probably by epithelial cells. Poger and Lamm (1974) have suggested that assembly of the secretory component and IgA probably occurs in the golgi apparatus or in the adjacent apical cytoplasm of epithelial cells. The secretory component is a single polypeptide chain containing carbohydrate (approximately 9 per cent) which becomes covalently bound to α chains in the Fc region of 80 per cent of secretory IgA molecules. Strong non-covalent interactions also help to stabilize the molecule. A schematic diagram of the secretory IgA molecule is shown in Figure 16. Both IgA1 and IgA2 are able to bind the secretory component, and there is no evidence of any structural difference between bound and free forms of the secretory component. The secretions of patients lacking IgA have been shown by South et al. (1966) to contain free secretory component in increased amounts. Such patients frequently have detectable secretory IgM instead of secretory IgA (Thompson, 1970).

2.4 Structure of Immunoglobulin M

2.4.1 Human Immunoglobulin M

IgM, also known as 19 S γ-globulin or γ-macroglobulin, occurs predominantly in man as a pentamer $(\mu_2 L_2)_5$ with a molecular weight of 950 000–1 000 000. However, both larger polymers and monomeric forms of IgM have been reported. The low molecular weight form (7 S IgM) is present at low concentrations in normal human serum, but at higher concentrations in patients with various immunological disorders (especially Waldenström's macroglobulinaemia, systemic lupus erythematosus, and ataxia telangiectasia).

The complete amino acid sequences of the μ chains from two Waldenström macroglobulins (Gal and Ou) have been reported (Watanabe et al., 1973; Putnam et al., 1973a, b) (see Figure 12), and the overall arrangement of polypeptide chains and disulphide bonds is illustrated in Figure 17. The macroglobulin is a pentamer of four-chain subunits, thus consisting of a total of ten light chains and ten heavy chains, plus one J chain. The μ chain has five intrachain disulphide loops or domains, each of similar size to the γ-chain domains. An allotypic marker on human IgM, designated Mm1, has been described by Wells et al. (1973), but little is known about its structural location. The μ chain is rich in carbohydrate having five oligosaccharide groups per chain (see Figure 17). These oligosaccharides are either simple or complex, but all contain glucosamine and are attached to asparagine residues in the obligatory sequence Asn–X–Ser/Thr. The function of these oligosaccharides has yet to be established

POLYPEPTIDE STRUCTURE OF HUMAN IgM

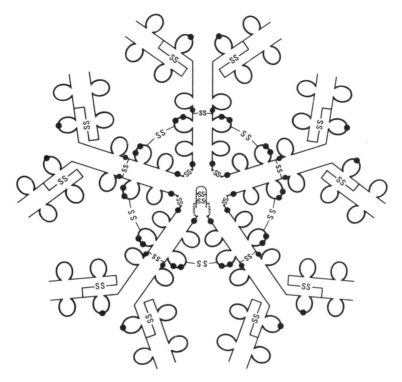

Figure 17 Schematic diagram of human IgM showing homology regions, carbohydrate side chains (●), and possible location of J chain (centre)

although it is known that they increase the solubility of the molecule and influence its conformation.

A single J chain occurs in each pentameric IgM molecule (Chapuis and Koshland, 1974) but the exact method of attachment remains open to discussion. Two different models of J-chain linkage have been proposed. In one the IgM monomer subunits are all disulphide-linked to the J chain which is held in a circular configuration by an intra-chain disulphide bridge. An alternative model envisages the J chain joined by disulphide bonds to two IgM monomers (a dimer clasp) or possibly disulphide bonded to one or both μ chains of a single monomer (a monomer clasp). The first (bracelet) model is now thought unlikely since recent evidence suggests that a single J chain is linked by disulphide bonds to the penultimate half-cystine residue of one or two μ chains only (Inman and Ricardo, 1974; Mestecky *et al.*, 1974). If this is so the J chain constitutes an asymmetric feature of polymeric IgM (see Figure 17) and it is suggested that the pentameric structure is stabilized through inter-subunit disulphide bridges between adjacent $C_\mu 3$ domains (Putnam *et al.*, 1973a).

30

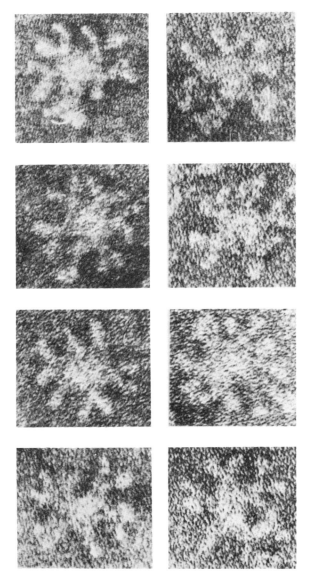

Figure 18 Electron micrographs of murine IgM (magnification × 660 000). Reproduced from Parkhouse *et al.* (1970), with permission

The IgM molecule has been a rewarding molecule for the electron micros-
copist. It has been shown that all the mammalian proteins studied have a
characteristic stellate structure in which the individual Fab arms of the five
subunits may sometimes be observed (see Figure 18).

The pentameric IgM molecule can be readily broken down to 7 S subunits by
mild reduction using, for example 0·015 M 2-mercaptoethylamine at neutral pH
(Morris and Inman, 1968). The 7 S subunits ($\mu_2 L_2$) are designated IgMs (where s
indicates subunit) and the ease with which they are obtained, in the absence of

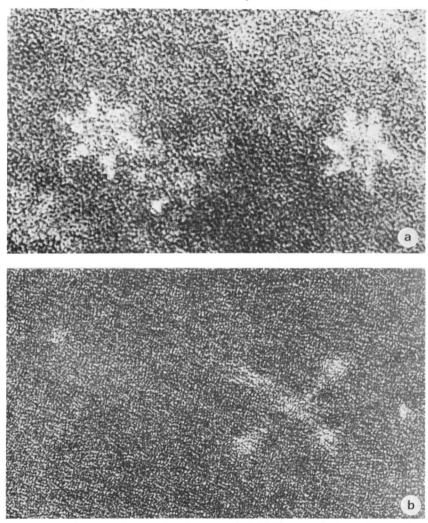

Figure 19 Electron micrographs of tetrameric IgM-like protein from the carp (*a*)
and hexameric IgM-like protein from the toad *Xenopus levi* (*b*). Micrographs by Dr.
E. Shelton and Dr. R. M. E. Parkhouse, respectively, and reproduced, with
permission, from Metzger (1970)

any dissociating agent, suggests that the stabilization of the pentamer is mainly through disulphide bridges. When 0·1–0·2 M 2-mercaptoethanol is used for dissociation, half-molecules (μL) sedimenting at 5 S may be obtained and these may then be used to prepare hybrid molecules (Frank and Humphrey, 1969; Solheim and Harboe, 1972). IgM can also be separated into its constituent heavy and light chains by conventional reduction procedures followed by alkylation and gel filtration in dissociating solvents (Cohen, 1963). Such procedures also release J chain and the separation of J and L chains requires an additional electrophoretic step.

Fragments of IgM analogous to the Fc, Fab, and $F(ab')_2$ of IgG may be produced by proteolytic cleavage with enzymes such as trypsin, papain, pepsin, and chymotrypsin—as reviewed by Metzger (1970). Treatment of the IgMs subunit with trypsin at 25° yields a Fab fragment (molecular weight 47 000), while treatment of the pentameric IgM with trypsin gives a $F(ab')_2$ fragment (molecular weight 114 000). Digestion of IgM with papain in the absence of thiols (Onoue et al., 1968) or with trypsin at 60° (Plaut and Tomasi, 1970) yields a pentameric $(Fc)_5\mu$ fragment (320 000–340 000) comprising the $C_\mu 3$ and $C_\mu 4$ domains of the μ chains.

2.4.2 Immunoglobulin M from Other Species

An IgM-like protein is present in the serum of nearly all vertebrates but its structure is variable. Whereas the molecule occurs in a pentameric form in mammals, birds, and reptiles, it exists as a hexamer in most amphibia, and as a tetramer in most teleosts (Figure 19). Marchalonis (1972) has shown that there are very few differences in amino acid composition between the high molecular weight immunoglobulins of lower vertebrates and the IgM of mammals. Moreover, the primitive IgM-like proteins resemble human IgM more closely than do human IgG or IgA.

Recent studies by Milstein et al. (1975) have shown that murine IgM has a subunit structure which closely resembles human IgM with the exception of the inter-subunit bonds in the two species. There is no disulphide bridge between adjacent $C_\mu 3$ domains in the mouse as in human IgM. The polymer appears to be bonded covalently solely through the penultimate cysteines of the $C_\mu 4$ domain (Figure 20).

2.5 Structure of Immunoglobulin D

IgD was first described by Rowe and Fahey (1965a, b) following investigations of an unusual myeloma protein. In normal human serum, the protein accounts for less than 1 per cent of the total plasma immunoglobulin and correspondingly only 1–3 per cent of cases of multiple myeloma involve this class.

Molecular weight studies of three IgD myeloma proteins (Leslie et al., 1971) indicate an average molecular weight of 69 000 for the δ chain and a molecular weight of 184 000 for the intact IgD molecule. This suggests that there may be five domains in the δ chain but this still has to be confirmed by sequence analysis.

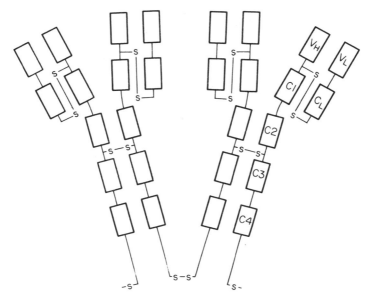

Figure 20 Possible arrangement of disulphide bridges in murine IgM.
Reproduced from Milstein *et al.* (1975), with permission

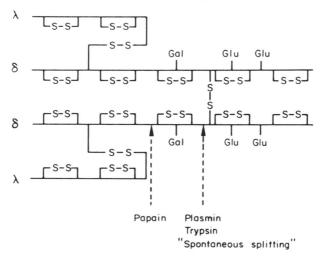

Figure 21 Schematic diagram of human IgD showing
possible location of oligosaccharide units and the single
inter-heavy chain disulphide bond. Reproduced from Stanworth and Turner (1973) with permission

Structural studies of IgD by Spiegelberg *et al.* (1970) have shown that the protein is unique among the human immunoglobulins in having only a single disulphide bridge between the two heavy chains (Figure 21). This immunoglobulin is rich in carbohydrate; the total amount present has been reported to range from 9 to 18 per cent. A striking finding is the presence of N-acetylgalactosamine (Jefferis *et al.*, 1975) which occurs also in IgA1 but no other immunoglobulin.

IgD is difficult to isolate from normal serum because it is present in low concentration. It is also liable to undergo spontaneous proteolysis by plasmin if ε-aminocaproate is not added to serum as an enzyme inhibitor. Spiegelberg *et al.* (1970) found that the protein is more susceptible to proteolysis than IgG1, IgG2, IgA, or IgM. Papain and trypsin both cleave the δ chains on the N-terminal side of the inter-heavy chain disulphide bridge, but trypsin cleaves at a point nearer to this bond to yield a larger Fab fragment (see Figure 21). Cleavage of the Fc_δ fragment with trypsin results in the loss of a hinge-region peptide (Spiegelberg *et al.*, 1970). Jefferis *et al.* (1975) have shown that, whereas the Fc_δ fragment contains all the carbohydrate of the intact molecule, the tFc_δ fragment lacks all the N-acetylgalactosamine and some ten residues of galactose. This suggests that the hinge region of IgD may be structurally similar to the hinge region of IgA1 (see p. 24).

2.6 Structure of Immunoglobulin E

Ishizaka *et al.* (1966) provided evidence for a fifth class of immunoglobulin having all the characteristics of homocytotropic or reaginic antibody. The concentration of the protein in normal serum is exceedingly low and further work on this immunoglobulin has been facilitated greatly by the identification of IgE myeloma proteins. A total of seven such proteins has now been described and studies on two of these (ND and PS) have provided most of the structural information about this class. Several aspects of this work have been reviewed by Bennich and Johansson (1971).

Electrophoretically IgE migrates in the fast γ region and is sedimented in the 8·0 S fraction following ultracentrifugation. The molecular weight of the whole molecule is about 188 000 and that of the isolated ε chain is about 72 500. The molecule exists as a four-chain unit with two light chains and two ε chains. The molecular weight of the ε chain without carbohydrate is about 61 000 which suggests that there are five structural domains in the molecule. Sequential analysis by Bennich and Bahr-Lindström has confirmed this.

When IgE is digested with papain, a 5 S Fc fragment with a molecular weight of 98 000 is released (Figure 22). This fragment which contains many of the IgE-specific determinants of the whole molecule and binds to the mast cell surface (see p. 000) also shares antigenic determinants (D1) with the $F(ab')_2$ fragment produced by pepsin (Bennich and Johansson, 1971). A fragment corresponding to the region of overlap has also been isolated and called Fc''.

The complete amino acid sequence of the ε chain of IgE (ND) was published by Bennich and Bahr-Lindström in 1974, and partial sequences of IgE (PS) are also

POLYPEPTIDE STRUCTURE OF HUMAN IgE

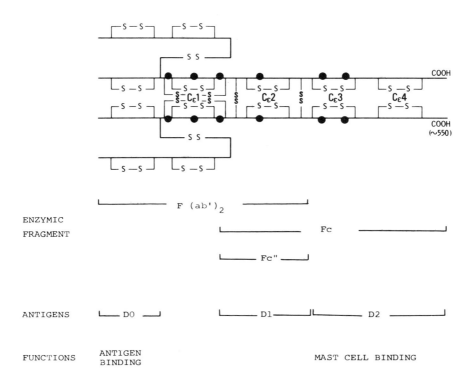

Figure 22 Schematic diagram of human IgE showing position of oligosaccharides (●). The location of various enzymic fragments, antigenic determinants, and biological activities are indicated. Data from Bennich and von Bahr-Lindström (1974)

available. Comparison of the C-region sequences from μ, γ, and α chains (see Figure 12) with the ε-chain sequence suggests that IgE has greatest homology with IgG (33 per cent).

IgE is unusual in having two inter-heavy chain disulphide bridges separated by a complete domain, that is, an inter-chain disulphide bridge between $C_\varepsilon 1$ and $C_\varepsilon 2$, and also between $C_\varepsilon 2$ and $C_\varepsilon 3$. Another feature which has been reported previously for rabbit IgG is the presence of an extra intra-chain disulphide bridge in the $C_\varepsilon 1$ homology region.

Since few human monoclonal IgE proteins have been described there is no evidence at present for the existence of any subclasses of IgE with possibly differing effector functions, nor is there any data on the structure of IgE from non-human species. However, the availability of monoclonal rat IgE will now make such studies feasible in this species (Bazin et al., 1974).

3 RELATIONSHIP BETWEEN STRUCTURE AND EFFECTOR FUNCTIONS OF IMMUNOGLOBULINS

3.1 Introduction

The primary function of immunoglobulins is, of course, to bind to antigen and the structure–activity relationships of the antigen-binding site are the subject of a separate chapter in this volume (Richards *et al.*, Chapter 2). This section will deal only briefly with this primary function and will consider solely the spectrum of antibody responses observed in immunoglobulin classes and subclasses. The remainder of Section 3 is concerned with the so-called 'secondary' manifestations of antigen–antibody interactions and the structural basis for such phenomena. The effector functions of the various proteins that constitute the human immunoglobulin system are summarized in Table 7.

Table 7 Major effector functions of human immunoglobulins

Immuno-globulin	Mean serum concen-tration (mg/ml)	Classical complement fixation	Alternate pathway comple-ment activation	Placental transfer	Binding to mono-nuclear cells	Binding to mast cells and basophils	Reactivity with staphy-lococcal protein A
IgG1	9	+ +	−	+	+	−	+
IgG2	3	+	−	+	−	−	+
IgG3	1	+ + +	−	+	+	−	−
IgG4	0·5	−	−*	+	−	(?)	+
IgM	1·5	+ + +	−	−	−	−	−
IgA1	3·0	−	+	−	−	−	−
IgA2	0·5	−	+	−	−	−	−
sIgA	0·05	−	−	−	−	−	−
IgD	0·03	−	−	−	−	−	−
IgE	0·00005	−	−*	−	−†	+ + +	−

* Aggregated molecules may activate complement by alternate pathway
† Human IgE has been reported to bind to macrophages

3.2 Antibody Populations and Immunoglobulin Classes

The nature of antibody populations is surprisingly variable and can range from essentially monoclonal responses (Braun *et al.*, 1969) to the widest possible heterogeneity involving all classes and subclasses. Many antibody responses, however, share certain common features such as an early IgM response (usually of low binding affinity) and a later, mainly IgG, response (usually of high binding affinity). In studies of human antibody responses to injected protein antigens such as tetanus toxoid, diphtheria toxoid, and thyroglobulin, it has been shown that antibody activity is present in all four IgG subclasses in approximately the same proportions as the subclass proteins themselves (Carrel *et al.*, 1972; Hay and Torrigiani, 1973; Spiegelberg, 1974). In contrast, some carbohydrate antigens give rise to a more restricted antibody response. For example, human antibody responses to injected dextrans and levans seem to be largely restricted to the IgG2 subclass (Yount *et al.*, 1968) and antibodies to the coagulation Factor VIII are found primarily in the IgG4 subclass (Anderson and Terry, 1968; Robboy *et al.*, 1970). In studies of IgG antibodies formed by grass pollen-allergic patients during immunotherapy, van der Giessen (1975) found that a relatively high proportion of grass pollen-specific antibodies belong to the IgG4 subclass. Other antibody responses appear to be restricted to two of the four subclasses. For example, anti-Rh antibodies (Natvig and Kunkel, 1973) are found in the IgG1 and IgG3 subclasses. Each of these restrictions may indicate that combinations between V and C-region genes are not totally random.

Injection is not, of course, the natural route of entry of an antigen. In studies of local responses to antigens introduced orally (polio virus—Ogra and Karzon, 1969) or intranasally (tetanus toxoid—Butcher *et al.*, 1975), it has been shown consistently that IgA is the predominant antibody class present in the local secretion, although in the case of a replicating antigen a specific antibody response also is elicited in all the major serum immunoglobulin fractions.

IgM antibody responses appear to be associated strongly with micro-organisms having a blood phase. This applies both to bacterial infections and protozoal parasites such as malaria and trypanosomiasis. The combined characteristics of good complement fixation, efficient agglutination, and predominantly intravascular location suggests that IgM plays a special role in eliminating micro-organisms from the blood stream. High levels of serum IgM in the newborn usually indicate an intrauterine infection such as rubella, syphilis, toxoplasmosis, or cytomegalovirus.

No major antibody function has yet been ascribed to IgD. Plasma cells secreting this immunoglobulin have been found in tonsillar and adenoid tissue, but occur rarely in spleen, peripheral lymphoid tissue, and the gut. Using sensitive techniques, IgD-specific binding to penicillin G (Gleich *et al.*, 1969), diphtheria toxoid (Heiner *et al.*, 1969), and insulin (Devey *et al.*, 1970) have been demonstrated at very low levels in selected sera. In both cord blood and blood from patients with chronic lymphocytic leukaemia IgD is the predominant class of surface immunoglobulin found on B lymphocytes and Rowe *et al.* (1973) have suggested that IgD functions as a lymphocytic receptor and is possibly involved in the induction of immunologic tolerance.

3.3 Membrane Transmission

Immunoglobulin transfer from a mother to her young occurs prenatally in man, postnatally in the pig, and during both phases in the rabbit, rat, and mouse. Prenatal transport of IgG occurs across placental membranes in man or yolk-sac membranes in the rat and mouse, whereas postnatal transport involves the passage of intact IgG, which is present in colostrum, across the membranes of the gut. In man, all four IgG subclasses appear to be able to cross the placenta (Wang *et al.*, 1970; Virella *et al.*, 1972), but in ruminants and the pig only the IgG1 subclass is absorbed through the gut.

Membrane transport has been investigated intensively by Brambell and coworkers who proposed a mechanism to explain their observations (Brambell *et al.*, 1960). According to this hypothesis serum proteins are taken up into pinocytotic vacuoles and IgG molecules become bound selectively through a specific receptor and are protected, whereas other protein molecules remain in the fluid phase and are catabolized. Thus, only IgG molecules, or a fraction of the total IgG in each vacuole, survive the journey across the placental membrane and are released intact on the foetal side. Whatever the mechanism involved, it is generally agreed that in all species it is both selective and saturable. For example, Waldmann *et al.* (1971) investigated the uptake and transport of radiolabelled proteins across segments of the neonatal rat duodenum. Only homologous IgG was transported at a high rate, and both IgG and Fc fragment were bound to surface membranes of purified enterocytes.

For obvious ethical reasons, there are little direct data on the transport of immunoglobulins and their fragments in man. However, Gitlin and coworkers (1964) injected labelled proteins into pregnant women volunteers at various stages of gestation and found that the Fc fragment of IgG was transported more rapidly to the foetus than was the Fab fragment, intact IgG, or any other protein. Work in other animals supports the view that the Fc region is critical, but there are as yet no data on which domain, C_H2 or C_H3, is the most important. For further details of the mechanism of membrane transmission see reviews by Waldmann and Strober (1969), and by Waldmann and Hemmings (1974).

3.4 Regulation of Catabolism

Each immunoglobulin class appears to be distinct metabolically with different synthetic and fractional catabolic rates (Table 8). The serum concentration of a particular protein is a reflection of the balance between synthesis and catabolism. For example, the synthetic rate for IgG (33 mg/Kg day^{-1}) is similar to that for IgA, but the serum concentration of the latter is much lower because of its higher fractional catabolic rate. The subclasses also differ one from another; thus IgG1, IgG2, and IgG4 have similar fractional catabolic rates (7 per cent of the intravenous pool degraded/day) and half lives of about 20 days, whereas IgG3 has a fractional catabolic rate of 17 per cent and a half life of seven days.

For IgG, the fractional catabolic rate is directly proportional to the serum concentration of this protein. Thus, in patients with G myeloma proteins, there is accelerated catabolism and the protein has a short half life, whereas in patients with sex-linked hypogammaglobulinaemia the fractional catabolic rate is reduced. For IgD and IgE, there appears to be an inverse relationship between the serum concentration and catabolic rate, whereas for IgM and IgA the fractional catabolic rate is independent of the serum concentration.

To explain the concentration–catabolism effects observed with IgG, Brambell *et al.* (1964) proposed a saturable protein-protection system specific for IgG molecules. According to this model, which is similar to that proposed to explain membrane transmission (see above), a constant fraction of the IgG molecules is isolated in a catabolic pool separate from the circulating protein pool (possibly within pinocytotic vacuoles). The site of such catabolism is not known; the liver,

Table 8 Metabolic characteristics of human immunoglobulins

Immuno-globulin	Half life (days)	Distribution (per cent intravascular)	Fractional catabolic rate (per cent intravascular pool catabolized/day)	Synthetic rate (mg/kg day^{-1})
IgG1	21 ⎫		7 ⎫	
IgG2	20 ⎪		7 ⎪	
IgG3	7 ⎬ 45		17 ⎬	33
IgG4	21 ⎭		7 ⎭	
IgM	10	80	8·8	3·3
IgA1	6 ⎫			
IgA2	6 ⎬	42	25	24
sIgA	—	—	—	—
IgD	3	75	37	0·4
IgE	2	50	71	0·002

gastrointestinal tract, and kidney have all been implicated, but the process may take place in the reticuloendothelial system all over the body. In any event, it is suggested that IgG molecules become attached to specific receptors from which they are returned to the circulation ultimately. The remaining unbound IgG molecules are degraded by proteolytic enzymes (cathepsins and neutral proteases).

The site of the IgG molecule which controls the rate of catabolism has been shown in several studies to reside in the Fc region (Waldmann *et al.*, 1971). The elimination of Fab and pFc' (equivalent to the C_H3 region) fragments of human IgG occurs rapidly in both man and the mouse. However, Fc fragments have a relatively long half life suggesting that the N-terminal half of the Fc region (equivalent to C_H2) is important in regulating the catabolic rate (Watkins *et al.*, 1971). This also is supported by the work of Dorrington and Painter (1974) who determined the half lives of the C_H2 and C_H3 fragments from human IgG1 injected intravenously into rabbits and compared them with the half lives of Fc, IgG1, and Fab in the same system. The C_H2 fragment, Fc fragment, and IgG have similar half lives of 60–70 hours, while the C_H3 and Fab fragments are eliminated much more rapidly; the half lives are between 16 and 17 hours.

Since Spiegelberg (cited by Waldmann and Hemmings, 1974) has reported that a monoclonal protein characterized as a half molecule of IgG (H + L) is eliminated rapidly from the circulation it appears that both heavy chains are required to provide the necessary conformation for normal catabolism. The present evidence therefore suggests that the dimeric C_H2 region of IgG is critical for the maintenance of a normal circulation time, although whether the mechanism of catabolism involves receptor binding with pinocytotic vacuoles, as envisaged by Brambell *et al.* (1960), is still far from clear.

3.5 Activation of Complement

The first step in the activation of complement by the classical pathway is the

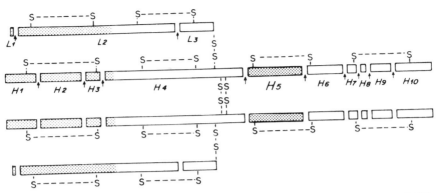

Figure 23 Schematic representation of the structure of a mouse myeloma IgG2a protein (MOPC 173) showing the localization of cyanogen bromide fragments produced by cleavage at the points indicated by the arrows. Peptide fragment (H5) has been shown to fix complement. Reproduced from Kehoe and Fougereau (1969), with permission of publisher

binding of the C1 subcomponent (C1q) to an IgG or IgM antibody. The association of this function with the Fc regions of these immunoglobulins was one of the first examples of the structural basis for the functional duality of antibody molecules (Müller-Eberhard and Kunkel, 1961; Augener et al., 1971).

The further localization of the complement-fixing site has, however, proved difficult. Kehoe and Fougereau (1969) isolated by cleavage with cyanogen bromide a fragment consisting of 60 amino acid residues from the C_H2 region of a monoclonal murine IgG2a protein (Figure 23). This fragment, when absorbed onto polystyrene latex particles, is able to fix guinea-pig complement, although on a molar basis only 3 per cent of the original activity remains.

Attempts to isolate biologically active subfragments from the Fc region of IgG by proteolytic digestion initially gave large fragments from the C_H3 region but much smaller peptides with molecular weights of less than 7000 from the C_H2 region; none of the latter has ever been shown to retain activity. However, Ellerson et al. (1972) were able to isolate a dimeric fragment of human IgG1 which corresponds closely to the C_H2 region plus the hinge region (residues 223–234). This was prepared by brief trypsin digestion of acid-treated Fc fragment and was characterized as a covalently bound dimer of the C_H2 region. In the C1q-binding assay of Augener et al. (1971), the fragment was found to have the same affinity for C1q as Fc when compared on a molar basis (Dorrington and Painter, 1974). Since reduced and alkylated β-microglobulin (a protein homologous to a single immunoglobulin domain) is able to interact with C1 in the same assay, it appears that little secondary or tertiary folding is required for the existence of an active C1-binding site.

Nevertheless hinge-region inter-heavy chain disulphide bridges are crucial for the binding of C1 by the intact IgG molecule. Isenman et al. (1975) have suggested that this effect is not related to the conformation of the active site itself but to the overall rigidity of the whole molecule and particularly the prevention of Fab regions from sterically hindering access of C1 to the site. These workers obtained further evidence in support of this hypothesis in comparative studies of C1 binding by IgG1 and IgG4 proteins and their Fc fragments. It is well established that IgG4 does not bind C1q (see Table 7) and it is surprising therefore that the Fc fragment of this subclass was found to be as active as the Fc fragment of IgG1. It is concluded that the structural features which allow C1 to interact with IgG are present in the IgG4 molecule but are not available in the presence of the Fab regions. It is possible that the heterogeneity of the IgG hinge regions (see Figure 8), with respect to position and number of inter-heavy chain disulphide bridges, is a critical factor in determining whether C1 binding occurs or not.

Further evidence that the C_H2 domain of IgG is involved in C1 fixation comes from work on an unusual fragment of rabbit IgG called Facb (Fragment antigen and complement binding). This is prepared by plasmin digestion of acid-treated IgG (Connell and Porter, 1971) and comprises the two Fab regions linked to the C_H2 region. The fragment lacks the C-terminal 108 amino acids of each heavy chain (that is the C_H3 region). This fragment has been found by Colomb and Porter (1975) to fix C1 by the classical complement pathway as efficiently as whole IgG which had been subjected to the same treatment with acid. Since the $F(ab')_2$ fragment is known not to fix complement, the activity of the Facb fragment again points to a C_H2 location for this function. It is of interest that the hinge region of rabbit IgG is not cleaved by plasmin presumably because the single lysine residue is adjacent to a proline residue. In contrast, human IgG1 has a lysine–threonine bond in the hinge region, and this is hydrolysed by plasmin.

IgM is, perhaps, a more important complement-fixing protein than IgG, but little is known about the structural localization of the complement-fixing site. Wolfenstein-Todel et al. (1973) showed that in the absence of antigen the pentameric $(Fc)_{5\mu}$ fragment is about 20 times more effective (on a molar basis) in complement fixation than the intact immunoglobulin. This suggests that the site is located in either the $C_\mu3$ or $C_\mu4$ domain and that it only becomes accessible after a conformational change brought about by interaction with antigen.

Hurst et al. (1974) studied the fixation of C1 by a monoclonal IgM protein and various fragments obtained by selective proteolysis and chemical degradation. A fragment (molecular weight 6800) from the C-terminal domain $C_\mu4$, and a fragment CNBr5, which contains the $C_\mu3$ and a portion of the $C_\mu4$ domain, were both found to bind C1 effectively. Subsequently, Hurst et al. (1975) characterized the $C_\mu4$ fragment which was obtained by limited tryptic cleavage of Fcμ—itself obtained by reduction of $(Fc)_{5\mu}$. The fragment consists of 24 residues on the N-terminal side of the $C_\mu4$ domain linked by a disulphide bridge to 32 residues on the C-terminal side of the loop, with 23 residues having been cleaved out of the centre of the disulphide loop (Figure 24). The activity of this fragment in a C1-fixation assay is decreased markedly following cleavage of the disulphide bridge, although the isolated A and B peptides do retain a limited ability to fix $\overline{C1}$. Hurst et al. (1975) have suggested that transient binding of C1 by the individual A and B

42

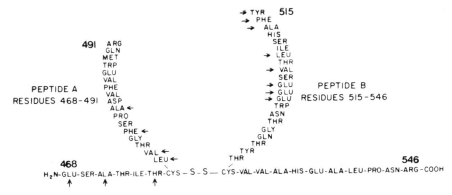

Figure 24 Primary amino acid sequence of the C_H4 fragment from human IgM wh has been shown to fix C1. Reproduced from Hurst *et al.* (1975) with permissic

peptide chains may be sufficient to activate C1, which in turn consumes

The J chain seems to play no role in classical complement fixation si pentameric IgM reassembled in its absence is only 25 per cent less effective in binding than the pentamer with J chain (Kownatzki and Drescher, 1ℂ Moreover, the $C_\mu4$ fragment studied by Hurst and coworkers (1975) appear to contain portions of J chain but to originate solely from the μ chain.

The alternative complement pathway, which does not involve C1, C4, or ι known to be activated by various immunoglobulin aggregates such as h IgA, guinea-pig IgG1, and ruminant IgG2. Isolated $F(ab')_2$ fragments froı guinea-pig IgG1 and IgG2 are able to activate the alternative pathway (Saı *et al.*, 1971). Similarly, rabbit $F(ab')_2$ fragments have been shown to cι Factor B (Spiegelberg and Götze, 1972). Since Fab fragments are not acti possible that a Factor B-binding site exists in the hinge region of these mc but no precise localization of such a site has been reported yet.

3.6 Interactions with Cell Membranes

3.6.1 *Macrophages and Monocytes*

Macrophage cytophilic antibodies were first described by Boyden and Sorkin (1960) who showed that such antibodies are capable of cellular fixation prior to their combination with antigen. Subsequently, Berken and Benacerraf (1966, 1968) have applied the term 'cytophilic' to those antibodies which become bound to macrophages after combination with antigen. These authors considered cytophilia to be a 'property of opsonizing antibody which provides the receptors which permit the binding of the antibody to the macrophage cell membrane in preparation for phagocytosis'. Other authors, notably Tizard (1969), have disputed this view and have claimed the existence of two distinct populations of antibody molecules. This aspect is considered further below.

Cytophilic binding to macrophages has been shown in rabbit (Boyden and Sorkin, 1960), guinea-pig (Berken and Benacerraf, 1966), and man (Lo Buglio *et al.*, 1967). In man, it has been shown that monocytic phagocytosis of erythrocytes coated with anti-Rh antibodies is inhibited by IgG1 and IgG3 myeloma proteins but not by IgG2 or IgG4 proteins (Huber and Fudenberg, 1968; Huber *et al.*, 1971). Similarly, Hay *et al.* (1972) showed that radiolabelled IgG1 and IgG3 myeloma proteins can bind strongly to the surface of the monocyte whereas IgG2 and IgG4 myeloma proteins bind poorly, if at all. Moreover, this binding can be inhibited both by fresh human serum and by soluble immune complexes.

Both Berken and Benacerraf (1966) and Lo Buglio *et al.* (1967) showed that the monocyte-binding activity of IgG is destroyed by digestion of the IgG with pepsin. Since these workers were studying residual $F(ab')_2$ fragments they considered that the results indicated an Fc location for the macrophage-binding site. In another study, Abramson *et al.* (1970) studied the capacity of various IgG fragments to inhibit rosette formation between anti-D-coated erythrocytes and human mononuclear cells. The Fc fragment was strongly inhibitory and the $F(ab')_2$ fragment weakly inhibitory. No inhibition was noted with Fab or with peptic peptides from the Fc region (including the pFc′ fragment). These authors concluded that the peptide portions of IgG which attach to mononuclear cells are located in the N-terminal half of the Fc fragment and require the integrity of inter-heavy chain disulphide bridge. In contrast, however, Yasmeen *et al.* (1973) showed that heterologous binding of human IgG to guinea-pig peritoneal macrophages is a function of the C_H3 domain but not of the N-terminal C_H2 domain. This was demonstrated both by a direct rosetting assay and by an indirect assay which measured the ability of various proteins to inhibit rosette formations between macrophages and erythrocytes coated with IgG. In the indirect assay, IgG, Fc, and C_H3 fragments were strongly inhibitory but C_H2 and Fab fragments are only weakly inhibitory. Using a homologous rosetting system of human monocytes and human erythrocytes coated with incomplete anti-D, Okafor *et al.* (1974) were able to study the inhibitory capacity of pFc′ fragments (equivalent to the C_H3 domain) obtained from all four IgG subclasses. Fragments from IgG1 and IgG3 myeloma proteins were significantly more inhibitory than fragments from IgG2 and IgG4 proteins, in agreement with the earlier work on intact immunoglobulin.

Recently, Ciccimarra *et al.* (1975) have reported that intact C_H3 and a peptide derived from it and provisionally located between residues 407–416 (Eu IgG1 numbering) are able to bind to human monocytes and also to inhibit rosette formation of antibody-coated erythrocytes with human monocytes. The amino acid sequences of IgG1 and IgG4 proteins are identical in this region except for residue 409 where an arginine/lysine substitution occurs. There are, however, no sequence data available for this region of IgG2 or IgG3 molecules to enable further comparisons to be made.

In contrast to the above workers, Holm *et al.* (1974) were unable to inhibit monocyte-mediated haemolysis with C_H3 fragments. These differences cannot at present be reconciled, but it is possible (Turner, 1974) that they relate to the different test system used. Furthermore, the observation of Dorrington and Painter (1974) that β_2-microglobulin is inhibitory in the monocyte-rosetting assay may indicate that cross-reactions occur between the heavy-chain domains.

The data of Hay *et al.* (1972) are consistent with the view first proposed by Berken and Benacerraf that the phagocyte-binding site of opsonizing antibodies is identical to the structure involved in cytophilic binding to macrophages. Thus, the inhibition of IgG1 and IgG3 binding to monocytes by soluble immune complexes is strikingly parallel to the inhibition by IgG1 and IgG3 of phagocytosis of opsonized red cells (Huber and Fudenberg, 1968). Furthermore, it was observed by Hay and coworkers (1972) that immune complexes are more effective than native immunoglobulins as inhibitors of IgG1 and IgG3 adherence. This may arise due to multipoint attachment of the complexes through several Fc regions giving much firmer binding than that established by the single Fc site of an individual IgG molecule.It seems probable, therefore, that uptake of antigen by phagocytic cells is much more likely to occur through an opsonizing antibody pathway than by the less efficient process of cytophilia. However, the site on the immunoglobulin molecule interacting with the macrophage membrane receptor may be identical in both processes.

Recently, Capron *et al.* (1975) have shown that rat IgE antibodies against *Schistosoma mansoni* antigens are able to bind to the schistosomules and also to adhere to peritoneal macrophages. The latter attachment was presumed to be Fc mediated, but further work is required to establish this unequivocally. A role of IgE-mediated macrophage adherence in schistosomiasis and other helminthic diseases is clearly an attractive possibility which would, if established, provide a rational biological function for this class of immunoglobulin.

3.6.2 Neutrophils

A receptor for IgG on the surface of human neutrophils was first reported by Messner and Jelinek (1970). Erythrocytes sensitized indirectly with antibacterial IgG antibodies, after passive sensitization with bacterial antigens, adhered to neutrophil monolayers and this adherence could be inhibited by whole IgG, IgG1, and IgG3 myeloma proteins, and by the Fc fragment but not by the Fab fragment.

Using an assay system based on the release of lysosomal constituents such as β-glucuronidase, Henson *et al.* (1972) concluded that, when aggregated, all four human IgG subclasses react with neutrophils. In addition, aggregated IgA1 and IgA2, but not IgM, IgD, or IgE, were found to be reactive. In a direct binding assay using $[^{125}I]$ immunoglobulins, Lawrence *et al.* (1975) found that neutrophils bind unaggregated myeloma proteins of the subclasses IgG1, IgG3, IgG4, IgA1, and IgA2. Furthermore, a preparation of secretory IgA was shown to bind. After aggregation with a rabbit $F(ab')_2$ anti-human Fab fragment reagent, neutrophils show increased binding of immunoglobulin of all classes.

The binding of IgA to neutrophils is the only known cytophilic property of this immunoglobulin class, although the biological significance of the observation remains to be evaluated. Since no significant cross-inhibition has been observed, it appears that the receptors for IgG and IgA on neutrophils are distinct but further work is clearly required in this field.

It seems likely that the IgG receptor interacting with phagocytic neutrophils is the same as that involved in monocyte/macrophage interactions, but the work of Messner and Jelinek (1970) with different rosetting systems suggests that the density of cell-surface receptors for IgG on neutrophils and monocytes differs.

3.6.3 Lymphocytes

B Lymphocytes usually have detectable surface immunoglobulin thought to be synthesized by the cell itself and T lymphocytes also appear to have small amounts of an IgM-like protein on their surface. In addition, there is evidence that human lymphocyte-like cells have receptors with specificity for both homologous and heterologous IgG (Brain and Marston, 1973; Frøland et al., 1973). Using inhibition of a rosette assay with IgG-sensitized indicator erythrocytes, Frøland et al. (1974) have studied the specificity of these receptors on so-called EA–RFC cells for various Ig subclasses and fragments. Both IgG1 and IgG3 inhibit strongly whereas IgG2 and IgG4 show only weak inhibition. No inhibition occurs using Fab or F(ab')$_2$ fragments, but the Fc fragment and the IgG3 Fch fragment (Fc plus the extended hinge region characteristic of IgG3) are strongly inhibitory. Partial reduction and alkylation reduces the inhibitory capacity of both fragments. The pFc' fragment of IgG (equivalent to the $C_\gamma 3$ region) is not inhibitory in this assay system, and the authors concluded that the $C_\gamma 2$ region is the probable molecular location of the receptor for lymphocyte-like cells. It seems very likely that the effector cells in antibody-dependent cytotoxicity (the K cells) are a subpopulation of these EA–RFC cells.

Lawrence et al. (1975) found that unaggregated IgG1 and IgG3 proteins bind to 'lymphocytes' but not IgG2, IgG4, IgA1, IgA2, IgM, IgE, IgD, or secretory IgA. However, unlike Frøland et al. (1974) who observed no differences following aggregation using a possibly different cell population, Lawrence and coworkers (1975) found that IgG of all subclasses and IgE are able to bind following aggregation with a rabbit F(ab')$_2$–anti-human Fab reagent. Preliminary studies with nylon fibre-purified T lymphocytes and B lymphocytes from a patient with chronic lymphocytic leukaemia suggest that both cell types have a receptor for IgG which is in agrement with other reports of IgG binding to B (Basten et al., 1972) and T lymphocytes of mouse (Anderson and Grey, 1974). Santana and Turk have shown that the binding of aggregated IgG to T cells requires large aggregates of greater than 200 S and that binding is temperature dependent (cited by Turner, 1974).

3.6.4 Basophils and Mast Cells

Immunoglobulin molecules with a capacity to bind to the membranes of basophils and mast cells are known as homocytotropic and have been recognized

46

Table 9 Properties of three major types of anaphylactic homocytotropic antibody in the guinea-pig

Property	IgE (Reagin)	IgG1	IgG2
Tissue sensitized	isologous	isologous	heterologous
Optimum sensitization time (hr)	50–80	2–4	2–4
Persistance in skin	4 weeks	1–2 days	1–2 days
Heat (56°, 30 min)	labile	stable	stable
C1q fixation	–	–	+

Modified from Stanworth (1970)

for many years. In several species, homocytotropic antibodies have been shown to be associated with two, or even three, distinct immunoglobulin classes (Table 9), but the most important biologically appears to be the reaginic (IgE) type (see reviews by Bennich and Johansson, 1971; Ishizaka and Ishizaka, 1971).

The concentration of IgE in serum is minute, and it is assumed that at any one time the bulk of the body pool is bound to the surface membranes of basophils and mast cells. The recent availability of rat myeloma IgE (Bazin *et al.* 1974) has permitted direct investigation of the interaction of IgE with rat basophilic leukaemic cells (Kulczycki *et al.*, 1974; Kulczycki and Metzger, 1974). From kinetic studies, it is clear that the interaction is described by the equation

$$\text{IgE} + \text{receptor} \underset{k_{-1}}{\overset{k_1}{\rightleftharpoons}} \text{receptor–IgE complex}$$

and that the association is first order both with regard to IgE and receptor concentrations. The reaction is specific, thus human IgE, heated rat IgE, rat IgG, rat IgA, and rat IgM do not bind, sites are saturable, and binding is reversible. The affinity constant ($K_A = k_1/k - 1$) has been calculated to be of the order of 6×10^9 M^{-1} and the number of binding sites per cell was found to be in the range 3×10^5 to more than 1×10^6.

An indirect estimation of k_A for the human IgE–basophil interation (Ishizaka *et al.*, 1973) gives values of 0.1–1.3×10^9 M^{-1} for 12 of 13 preparations and 1.2×10^{10} M^{-1} for the other. In the same study, the number of receptors per cell was found to be in the range 3×10^4–8.5×10^4, although such numbers should be intepreted with caution since they appear to be a variable characteristic of different cell types (Kulczycki and Metzger, 1974) and may also vary with the metabolic state of the cell.

The structural location of the mastcell-binding site of IgE is still under investigation and at the time of writing has not been localized more precisely than the $C_\varepsilon 3$–$C_\varepsilon 4$ regions. Bennich and von Bahr-Lindstrom (1974) have suggested that the binding of an IgE molecule to a mast cell or basophil cell surface membrane may involve two distinct sites in the $C_\varepsilon 3$–$C_\varepsilon 4$ regions. One type of site, which they have termed 'primary', has a recognition function, interacts with a membrane receptor on the basophil or mast cell, and may be located in the $C_\varepsilon 4$

domain. A 'secondary' binding site is proposed also, which may be present in either domain, shows no particular cell specificity, and is capable of interacting with any cell membrane.

It is well established that the ability of IgE to bind to mast cells and basophils is lost following heat treatment at 56° for 30 minutes. The structural changes induced by such treatment were studied by Dorrington and Bennich (1973) using circular dichroism and ultraviolet absorption difference spectra. It was found that intact IgE showed changes in both the aromatic side-chain and peptide-bond spectral regions, which were only partially reversible on cooling. Similar studies were performed with the $F(ab')_2$, Fc″, and Fc fragments of IgE (see Figure 22); the conformational changes induced in $F(ab')_2$ and Fc″ fragments were fully reversible. Furthermore, antigenic determinants known to be located in the Fc″ region were unaffected by prolonged exposure to heat. These studies indicate that the irreversible thermal effects are restricted to the two C-terminal domains, one or both of which are known to carry the cytotropic site.

Recently, Hamburger (1975) has reported that a pentapeptide (Asp-Ser-Asp-Pro-Arg) corresponding in sequence to amino acid residues 320–324 (that is adjacent to the inter-heavy chain disulphide bridge between $C_\varepsilon 2$ and $C_\varepsilon 3$) is able to inhibit *in vivo* passive transfer of IgE-mediated sensitivity in the Prausnitz–Küstner test. Whether or not this represents the mast cell binding site of the IgE molecule is a controversial issue and the focus of much current research.

As stressed earlier there exists, in several species, a second type of homocytotropic antibody which is usually of IgG-type and which characteristically sensitizes homologous tissues for short periods. Established examples of this type of antibody are IgGa of rat, IgG1 of guinea-pig, IgG1 of mouse, and IgS of sheep. Studies of rat homocytotropic antibodies by Bach *et al.* (1971) suggest that IgE and IgGa compete for the same cell receptor although the affinity of IgG is much lower than that of IgE.

Man also appears to have a weak cell-binding, heat-stable, mercaptoethanol-resistant homocytotropic IgG antibody capable of passively sensitizing human or primate skin for two to four hours (Malley and Perlman, 1966; Parish, 1974). An antibody with similar properties to this so-called 'short-term sensitizing antibody' (IgG S–TS) has been described in subjects sensitive to horse serum (Terr and Bentz, 1965) and in asthmatic patients unresponsive to disodium cromoglycate (Bryant *et al.*, 1973). There is no direct evidence that IgG S–TS belongs to any of the known subclasses, although Stanworth and Smith (1973) have reported that an IgG4 myeloma protein is able to block the binding of human IgE to baboon mast cells.

A biologically unimportant homocytotropic antibody activity can be demonstrated in human, rabbit, and mouse IgG. Each of these immunoglobulins can sensitize heterologous (guinea-pig) skin for reverse passive cutaneous anaphylaxis reactions (Ovary, 1960). The subclasses involved—IgG1, IgG3, and IgG4 of man, and IgG2a of mouse and rat (Ovary *et al.*, 1965; Terry, 1966)—do not sensitize isologous skin and are thus generally distinct from the short-term sensitizing IgG homocytotropic antibodies.

3.7 Reactivity with Staphylococcal Protein A

In 1966, Forsgren and Sjöquist reported that a cell-wall protein, called protein A isolated from *Staphylococcus aureus* is able to bind the Fc region of human IgG. This was confirmed by Kronvall (1967) and extended to the IgG of other species, including rabbit (Forsgren and Sjöquist, 1967), guinea-pig IgG1 and IgG2 (Forsgren, 1968), and mouse IgG (Kronvall *et al.*, 1970*a*).

In man, anti-protein A reactivity is confined to the IgG1, IgG2, and IgG4 subclasses (Kronvall and Williams, 1969), while in the mouse IgG2a, IgG2b, and IgG3 are reactive but not IgG1 (Kronvall *et al.*, 1970*a*). Human IgA and IgM were found to be unreactive (Kronvall *et al.*, 1970*c*). In a separate study, a single IgD and a single IgE myeloma protein were also unreactive (Kronvall *et al.*, 1970*a*). (*Note added in proof:* Recent work (Saltvedt and Harboe, 1976) has shown that proteins of the human IgA2 subclass react with staphylococci and that some IgM proteins (provisionally designated IgM2) are also reactive.)

Kronvall and Frommel (1970) used a procedure involving the inhibition of precipitation to show that protein A reactivity is a property of the Fc fragment and heavy chains but not of F(ab′)$_2$, Fab, Fc′, and pFc′ fragments, or of light chains. This suggests that protein A binding is yet another function of the C_H2 domain but this remains to be demonstrated in a direct-binding assay.

Kronvall *et al.* (1970*b*) measured the equilibrium constant of two different IgG myeloma proteins for staphylococcal protein A and found both to be about $4 \times 10^7 \, M^{-1}$. In the same study, the number of protein A residues was estimated to be 80 000/organism, which is four times the density of the blood group A antigen on erythrocytes.

The biological importance of protein A binding is not yet fully understood, but several studies point to a possible involvement in non-immune complement activation. For example, protein A–IgG complexes can fix guinea-pig complement (Sjöquist and Stålenheim, 1969; Kronvall and Gewurz, 1970; Stålenheim and Malmheden-Eriksson, 1971) and also complement from fresh human, pig, and dog sera (Kronvall and Gewurz, 1970). Also, Kronvall and Gewurz (1970) have suggested that protein A is able to bring IgG molecules into the close spatial proximity necessary for activation of C1 esterase. Both dimerization of IgG by protein A and larger structures due to secondary aggregation may produce complement-activating complexes. This suggestion is supported further by the studies of Stålenheim and Castensson (1971) who found that when protein A is added to human serum C3 is converted to C3a and C3b. However, neither protein A nor aggregates of protein A and IgG can convert purified C3. The most probable explanation of these observations is that protein A reacts with the Fc region of IgG and that C1 is then activated by fixation to the protein A–IgG complex. Thus, according to this view the protein A–IgG complex initiates complement fixation by the classical pathway in much the same way as an ordinary antigen–antibody complex.

3.8 Interaction with Rheumatoid Factors

Rheumatoid factors are a group of serum proteins first described by Waaler

(1940) and by Rose *et al.* (1948). Subsequently, they were characterized as IgM antibodies reacting with antigenic determinants of both human and foreign species IgG (Hobson and Gorrill, 1952; Grubb, 1956; Waller and Vaughan, 1956). These antigenic determinants have been shown by several investigators to be located in the Fc region of the molecule—see for example Franklin (1961), Osterland *et al.* (1963), and Henney and Stanworth (1964)—but, although some authors have taken the view that they arise after conformational alteration of IgG, there is no unequivocal evidence to support this.

Several of the Gm allotypic antigens interact with rheumatoid factors and were, in many cases, first described and defined using serum from patients with rheumatoid arthritis (Grubb and Laurell, 1956; Harboe, 1959; Natvig, 1966). More recently, the nG1m(a) and γ_4 non-a antigens, which are antithetic to G1m(a), and the nG3m(b^1) antigen, which is antithetic to G3m(b^1), have been shown to interact with appropriate rheumatoid factors (Gaarder and Natvig, 1972; Natvig *et al.*, 1972). The nG1m(a) and nG3m(b^1) antigens are shared by several subclasses and behave as both allotypic and isotypic antigens. The isotypic Ga antigen (Allen and Kunkel, 1966; Gaarder and Natvig, 1970) is shared by the IgG1, IgG2, and IgG4 subclasses and is probably the most important of all the antigens interacting with rheumatoid factors. It is unrelated apparently to either the G3m(g) or G3m(b^1) antigens which are present on IgG3 molecules. Furthermore, the latter antigens probably occupy different molecular locations in the γ_3 chain since there are antithetic nG3m(g) and nG3m(b^1) markers for each allotype.

A provisional localization of the antigens interacting with serologically defined rheumatoid factors has been achieved using various proteolytic fragments (Natvig and Turner, 1970; Natvig *et al.*, 1972). As shown in Table 10 all the

Table 10 Molecular location of isotypic and allotypic antigens of human IgG known to interact with appropriate rheumatoid factors

Immunoglobulin subclass and allotype			Homology region		
			C_H2	C_H3	
IgG1	G1m(ax)	Ga	nG3m(b^1)	G1m(a)	G1m(x)
IgG1	G1m(f)	Ga	nG3m(b^1)	nG1m(a)	
IgG2	G2m(n +)	Ga	nG3m(b^1)	nG1m(a)	
IgG2	G2m(n −)	Ga	nG3m(b^1)	nG1m(a)	
IgG3	G3m(g)	G3m(g)	nG3m(b^1)	nG1m(a)	
IgG3	G3m(b)		G3m(b^1)	nG1m(a)	
IgG4	a	Ga	γ_4 non-a		
IgG4	b	Ga	γ_4 non-a		

antigens are in the Fc region and the eight known specificities appear to be determined by amino acid substitutions in five antigenic regions. Using pFc′ fragments (equivalent to C_H3 fragments) from each allotypic variant of the four subclasses in a haemagglutination-inhibition assay system, it was possible to demonstrate the presence of the antithetic G1m(a), nG1m(a) and γ_4 non-a antigens in the C_H3 region. From earlier sequence studies, it appears that these

Table 11 Amino acid sequences associated with three antigens interacting with rheumatoid factors

Subclass	Antigen	Sequence number			
		355	356	357	358
IgG1	G1m(a)	Arg	*Asp*	Glu	*Leu*
IgG1 G1m(f) ⎫ IgG2 ⎬ IgG3 ⎭	nG1m(a)	Arg	Glu	Glu	Met
IgG4	γ_4 non-a	*Gln*	Glu	Glu	Met

antigens are specified by amino acid residues located between residues 355 and 358 of the γ chain (following the Eu numbering of Edelman *et al.*, 1969). The sequences and associated antigens are given in Table 11.

There is evidence from studies using antiglobulins obtained from sensitized healthy individuals that the expression of each of these antigens requires the presence of a non-correlative determinant located near the C-terminus of the γ chain (Turner *et al.*, 1969, 1972). Work with a rheumatoid factor interacting with G1m(a) suggests a similar requirement for this antigen-antibody system (Okafor and Turner, 1974). Whether this determinant is actually part of these antigenic sites or merely influences their conformation is not clear.

The G1m(x) antigen also is known to be present in the C_H3 region but there are insufficient sequence data available to permit a more precise localization. By virtue of the failure of pFc' fragments to inhibit the binding of appropriate specific rheumatoid factors the following antigens are presumed to be located in the C_H2 domain: the antithetic G3m(b^1) and nG3m(b^1) antigens; the G3m(g) antigen; and the Ga antigen. With the exception of G3m(g), which may be specified by residue 296 (see Table 6), there are no sequence data for these antigens.

Earlier studies (Normansell, 1970, 1971) have indicated a low binding affinity between a rheumatoid factor of undefined specificity and both native and aggregated IgG. More recently, Steward *et al.* (1973) have measured the binding affinities of rheumatoid factors interacting with the G1m(a), G1m(x), nG1m(a), and γ_4 non-a antigens using single antigen systems of appropriate, isolated C_H3 fragments. All the rheumatoid factors studied show specific binding with the fragments possessing the homologous antigen and the binding affinities of these rheumatoid factors are low—between 10^4 and 10^5 M^{-1}. A similar value has been obtained by Dissanyake *et al.* (unpublished results) using the isolated Fab fragment of an IgM rheumatoid factor and either native or aggregated IgG. The impressive superior reactivity of aggregated IgG with rheumatoid factors is yet another example of the biological amplification effect which is possible when multivalent attachment occurs.

3.9 Future Perspectives

In the preceding sections the evidence for the location of various IgG effector

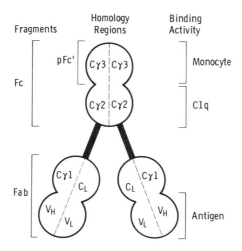

Figure 25 Schematic diagram of human IgG showing homology regions, enzymic fragments, and the location of various biological activities

functions has been reviewed briefly and some data are summarized in Figure 25. It seems likely that in the immediate future the precise localization of the rheumatoid factor antigens will be the most readily achieved since these are antigenic determinants which correlate with specific amino acid sequences found within a single allotype or an isotype with an antithetic marker.

In contrast, a full understanding of the molecular configuration required for binding C_{1q} or for the interaction with cell-membrane receptors will require considerable advances in the X-ray crystallography field. At the present time no effector function site is mapped within the three-dimensional structure in the same detail as the antibody combining site. The recent report (Colman *et al.*, 1976) of the structure of a whole IgG molecule at 0·5 nm resolution is the best source of data available for the Fc region and suggests that there is a degree of flexibility in this region. This is not incompatible with the view that allosteric changes may occur in immunoglobulins following antigen binding to expose a C_{1q} binding site (in the case of IgG and IgM) or perhaps initiate mast cell degranulation (in the case of IgE).

The biological activity of the cell-binding immunoglobulins may prove the most difficult to dissect. The possible involvement of two sites has been proposed in connection with IgE–mast cell interactions (see pp. 46–47) (Stanworth, 1973; Bennich and Bahr-Lindstrom, 1974), and may be applicable to other Ig–cell systems. Cell binding may involve a site in a single domain or it may, conceivably, require co-operation between adjacent domains. This could explain some of the discrepancies observed in the case of monocyte binding.

Although there is at present a dearth of information on the structural basis of immunoglobulin effector functions it is to be expected that current interests in

52

membrane biochemistry and cell-triggering phenomena will act as a stimulus to further investigations in this area of immunochemistry.

REFERENCES

Abramson, N., Gelfand, E. W., Jandl, J. H., and Rosen, F. S. (1970). *J. Exp. Med.*, **132**, 1207.
Allen, J. C., and Kunkel, H. G. (1966). *Arth. Rheumat.* **9**, 758.
Amzel, L. M., Chen, B. L., Phizackerly, R. P., Poljak, R. J., and Saul, F. (1974). In *Progress in Immunology II*, Vol. I, (Brent, L., and Holborow, J., eds.), North Holland Publishing Co., Amsterdam, p. 85.
Anderson, C. L., and Grey, H. M. (1974). *J. Exp. Med.*, **139**, 1175.
Anderson, J. R., and Terry, W. D. (1968). *Nature (Lond.)*, **217**, 174.
Atwell, J. L., and Marchalonis, J. J. (1975). *J. Immunogenetics*, **1**, 391.
Atwell, J. L., and Marchalonis, J. J. (1976). In *Comparative Immunology*, (Marcholonis, J. J., ed.), Blackwell, Oxford. p. 276
Augener, W., Grey, H. M., Cooper, N. R., and Müller-Eberhard, H. J. (1971). *Immunochemistry*, **8**, 1011.

Bach, M. K., Bloch, K. J., and Austen, K. F. (1971). *J. Exp. Med.*, **133**, 752.
Baglioni, C., Alescio-Zonta, L., Cioli, D., and Carbonara, A. (1966). *Science, N.Y.*, **152**, 1517.
Basten, A., Miller, J. F. A. P., Spent, J., and Pye, J. (1972). *J. Exp. Med.*, **135**, 610.
Bazin, H., Querinjean, P., Beckers, A., Heremans, J. F., and Dessy, F. (1974). *Immunology*, **26**, 713.
Bennich, H., and Johansson, S. G. O. (1971). *Adv. Immunol.*, **13**, 1.
Bennich, H., and von Bahr-Lindstrom, H. (1974). In *Progress in Immunology II*, Vol. I, (Brent, L., and Holborow, J., eds.), North Holland Publishing Co., Amsterdam, p. 49.
Berken, A., and Benacerraf, B. (1966). *J. Exp. Med.*, **123**, 119.
Berken, A., and Banacerraf, B. (1968). *J. Immunol.*, **100**, 1219.
Bernier, G. M., Tominaga, K., Easley, C. W., and Putnam, F. W. (1965). *Biochemistry*, **4**, 2072.
Boyden, S. V., and Sorkin, E. (1960). *Immunology*, **3**, 272.
Brain, P., and Marston, R. H. (1973). *Eur. J. Immunol.*, **3**, 6.
Brambell, F. W. R., Hemmings, W. A., and Morris, I. G. (1964). *Nature (Lond.)*, **203**, 1352.
Brambell, F. W. R., Hemmings, W. A., Oakley, C. L., and Porter, R. R. (1960). *Proc. Roy. Soc. Ser. B.*, **151**, 478.
Braun, D. G., Eichmann, K., and Krause, R. M. (1969). *J. Exp. Med.*, **129**, 809.
Bryant, D. H., Burns, M. W., and Lazarus, L. (1973). *Brit. Med. J.*, *iv*, 589.
Butcher, B. T., Salvaggio, J. E., and Leslie, G. A. (1975). *Clin. Allergy*, **1**, 33.

Capra, J. D., and Kindt, T. J. (1975). *Immunogenetics*, **1**, 417.
Capron, A., Dessaint, J.-P., Capron, M., and Bazin, H. (1975). *Nature (Lond.)*, **253**, 474.
Carrel, S., Morell, A., Skvaril, F., and Barandun, S. (1972). *FEBS Letters*, **19**, 305.
Chapuis, R. M., and Koshland, M. E. (1974). *Proc. Nat. Acad. Sci., U.S.A.*, **71**, 657.
Chodirker, W. B., and Tomasi, T. B. (1963). *Science, N.Y.*, **142**, 1080.
Ciccimarra, F., Rosen, F. S., and Merler, E. (1975). *Proc. Nat. Acad. Sci., U.S.A.*, **72**, 2081.
Cohen, S. (1963). *Biochem. J.*, **89**, 334.
Colman, P. M., Deisenhofer, J., Huber, R., and Palm, W. (1976). *J. Mol. Biol.*, **100**, 257.
Colomb, M., and Porter, R. R. (1975). *Biochem. J.*, **145**, 177.

Connell, G. E., and Porter, R. R. (1971). *Biochem. J.*, **124**, 53P.

De Préval, X., Pink, J. R. L., and Milstein, C. (1970). *Nature (Lond.)*, **228**, 930.
Devey, M., Carter, D., Sanderson, C. J., and Coombs, R.R.A. (1970). *Lancet, ii*, 1280.
Dorrington, K. J., and Bennich, H. (1973). *J. Biol. Chem.*, **248**, 8378.
Dorrington, K. J., and Painter, R. H. (1974). In *Progress in Immunology II*, Vol. I, (Brent, L., and Holborow, J., eds.), North Holland Publishing Co., Amsterdam, p. 75.
Dorrington, K. J., and Rockey, J. H. (1970). *Biochim. Biophys. Acta*, **200**, 584.
Dreyer, W. J., and Bennett, J. C. (1965). *Proc. Nat. Acad. Sci., U.S.A.*, **54**, 864.

Edelman, G. M. (1970). *Biochemistry*, **9**, 3197.
Edelman, G. M., Cunningham, B. A., Gall, W. E., Gottlieb, P. D., Rutishauser, U., and Waxdal, M. J. (1969). *Proc. Nat. Acad. Sci., U.S.A.*, **63**, 78,
Edelman, G. M., and Gall, W. E. (1969). *Ann. Rev. Biochem.*, **38**, 415.
Edelman, G. M., and Gally, J. A. (1962). *J. Exp. Med.*, **116**, 207.
Edelman, G. M., and Poulik, M. D. (1961). *J. Exp. Med.*, **113**, 861.
Ellerson, J. R., Yasmeen, D., Painter, R. H., and Dorrington, K. J. (1972). *FEBS Letters*, **24**, 318.
Edmundson, A. B., Ely, K. R., Girling, R. L., Abola, E. E., Schiffer, M, and Westholm, F. A. (1974). In *Progress in Immunology II*, Vol. I, (Brent, L., and Holborow, J., eds.), North Holland Publishing Co., Amsterdam, p. 103.

Feinstein, A., and Rowe, A. J. (1965). *Nature (Lond.)*, **205**, 147.
Feinstein, D., and Franklin, E. C. (1966). *Nature (Lond.)*, **212**, 1496.
Fleischman, J. B., Pain, R., and Porter, R. R. (1961). *Archs Biochem. Biophys.*, Suppl. 1, 174.
Forsgren, A. (1968). *J. Immunol.*, **100**, 921.
Forsgren, A., and Sjöquist, J. (1966). *J. Immunol.*, **97**, 822.
Forsgren, A., and Sjöquist, J. (1967). *J. Immunol.*, **99**, 19.
Frangione, B., and Milstein, C. (1968). *J. Mol. Biol.*, **33**, 893.
Frangione, B., and Wolfenstein-Todel, C. (1972). *Proc. Nat. Acad. Sci., U.S.A.*, **69**, 3673.
Frank, M. M., and Humphrey, J. H. (1969). *Immunology*, **17**, 237.
Franklin, E. C. (1961). *Proc. 10th Int. Congr. Rheumatol.*, **2**, 804.
Frøland, S. S., Michaelsen, T. E., Wisløff, F., and Natvig, J. B. (1974). *Scand. J. Immunol.*, **3**, 509.
Frøland, S. S., Natvig, J. B., and Wisløff, F. (1973). *Scand. J. Immunol.*, **2**, 83.

Gaarder, P. I., and Natvig, J. B. (1970). *J. Immunol.*, **105**, 928.
Gaarder, P. I., and Natvig, J. B. (1972). *J. Immunol.*, **108**, 617.
Gitlin, D., Kumate, J., Urrusti, J., and Morales, C. (1964). *J. Clin. Invest.*, **43**, 1938.
Gleich, G. J., Bieger, R. C., and Stankievic, R. (1969). *Science, N.Y.*, **165**, 606.
Grabar, P., and Williams, C. A. Jr. (1953). *Biochim. Biophys. Acta*, **10**, 193.
Grey, H. M., Abel, C. A., Yount, W. J., and Kunkel, H. G. (1968). *J. Exp. Med.*, **128**, 1223.
Grey, H. M., Hirst, J. W., and Cohn, M. (1971). *J. Exp. Med.*, **133**, 289.
Grubb, R. (1956). *Acta path. microbiol. scand.*, **39**, 195.
Grubb, R., and Laurell, A. B. (1956). *Acta path. microbiol. scand.*, **39**, 390.

Hamburger, R. (1975). *Science, N.Y.*, **189**, 389.
Harboe, M. (1959). *Acta path microbiol scand.*, **47**, 191.
Hay, F. C., and Torrigiani, G. (1973). *Clin. Exp. Immunol.*, **15**, 517.
Hay, F. C., Torrigiani, G., and Roitt, I. M. (1972). *Eur. J. Immunol.*, **2**, 257.
Heiner, D. C., Saha, A., and Rose, B. (1969). *Fed. Proc.*, **28**, 766.
Henney, C. S., and Stanworth, D. R. (1964). *Nature (Lond.)*, **201**, 511.
Henson, P. M., Johnson, H. B., and Spiegelberg, H. L. (1972). *J. Immunol.*, **109**, 1182.

54

Heremans, J. F. (1959). *Clin. Chim. Acta*, **4**, 639.
Hill, R. L., Delaney, R., Lebovitz, H. E., and Fellows, R. E. (1966). *Proc. Roy. Soc., Ser. B.*, **166**, 159.
Hilschmann, N., and Craig, L. C. (1965). *Proc. Nat. Acad. Sci., U.S.A.*, **53**, 1403.
Hobson, D., and Gorrill, R. H. (1952). *Lancet, i*, 389.
Holm, G., Engvall, E., Hammarström, S., and Natvig, J. B. (1974). *Scand. J. Immunol.*, **3**, 173.
Huber, H., Douglas, S. D., Nusbacher, J., Kochwa, S., and Rosenfield, R. E. (1971). *Nature (Lond.)*, **229**, 419.
Huber, H., and Fudenberg, H. H. (1968). *Int. Archs Allergy*, **34**, 18.
Hurst, M. M., Volanakis, J. E., Hester, R. B., Stroud, R. M., and Bennett, J.C. (1974). *J. Exp. Med.*, **140**, 1117.
Hurst, M. M., Volanakis, J. E., Stroud, R. M., and Bennett, J. C. (1975). *J. Exp. Med.*, **142**, 1322.

Inman, F. P., and Ricardo, M. J. (1974). *J. Immunol.*, **112**, 229.
Isenman, D. E., Dorrington, K. J., and Painter, R. H. (1975). *J. Immunol.*, **114**, 1726.
Ishizaka, K., and Ishizaka, T. (1971), *Clin. Allergy*, **1**, 9.
Ishizaka, K., Ishizaka, T., and Hornbrook, M. M. (1966). *J. Immunol.*, **97**, 75.
Ishizaka, T., Soto, C. S., and Ishizaka, K. (1973). *J. Immunol.*, **111**, 500.

Jefferis, R., Butwell, A. J., and Clamp, J. R. (1975). *Clin. Exp. Immunol.*, **22**, 311.

Kehoe, J. M., and Fougereau, M. (1969). *Nature (Lond.)*, **224**, 1212.
Köhler, H., Shimizu, A., Paul, C., Moore, V., and Putnam, F. W. (1970). *Nature (Lond.)*, **227**, 1318.
Kownatzki, E., and Drescher, M. (1973). *Clin. Exp. Immunol.*, **15**, 557.
Kratzin, H., Altevogt, P., Ruban, E., Kortt, A., Staroscik, K., and Hilschmann, N. (1975). *Hoppe-Seyler's Z. Physiol. Chem.*, **356**, 1337.
Kronvall, G. (1967). *Acta. path. microbiol. scand.*, **69**, 619.
Kronvall, G., and Frommel, D. (1970. *Immunochemistry*, **7**, 124.
Kronvall, G., and Gewurz, H. (1970). *Clin. Exp. Immunol.*, **7**, 211.
Kronvall, G., Grey, H. M., and Williams, R. C., Jr. (1970a). *J. Immunol.*, **105**, 1116.
Kronvall, G., Quie, P. G., and Williams, R. C., Jr. (1970b). *J. Immunol.*, **104**, 273.
Kronvall, G., Seal, U.S., Finstad, J., and Williams, R. C., Jr. (1970c). *J. Immunol.*, **104**, 140.
Kronvall, G., and Williams, R. C., Jr. (1969). *J. Immunol.*, **103**, 828.
Kulczycki, A., Isersky, C., and Metzger, H. (1974). *J. Exp. Med.*, **139**, 600.
Kulczycki, A., and Metzger, H. (1974). *J. Exp. Med.*, **140**, 1676.
Kunkel, H. G., and Prendergast, R. A. (1966). *Proc. Soc. Exp. Biol. Med.*, **122**, 910.

Lawrence, D. A., Weigle, W. O., and Spiegelberg, H. L. (1975). *J. Clin. Invest.*, **55**, 368.
Leslie, G. A., Clem, L. W., and Rowe, D. (1971). *Immunochemistry*, **8**, 565.
Lo Buglio, A. F., Cotran, R. S., and Jandl, J. H. (1967). *Science, N.Y.*, **158**, 1582.

Malley, A., and Perlman, F. (1966). *Proc. Soc. Exp. Biol. Med.*, **122**, 152.
Marchalonis, J. J. (1972). *Nature, New Biol.*, **236**, 84.
Messner, R. P., and Jelinek, J. (1970). *J. Clin. Invest.*, **49**, 2165.
Mestecky, J., Schrohenloher, R. E., and Kulhavy, R. (1974). *Fed. Proc.*, **33**, 747.
Mestecky, J., Schrohenloher, R. E., Kulhavy, R., Wright, G. P., and Tomana, M. (1974). *Proc. Nat. Acad. Sci., U.S.A.*, **71**, 544.
Metzger, H. (1970). *Adv. Immunol.*, **12**, 57.
Michaelsen, T. E. (1973). *Scand. J. Immunol.*, **2**, 523.
Milstein, C. (1966). *Nature (Lond.)*, **209**, 370.

Milstein, C., and Svasti, J. (1971). In *Progress in Immunology*, Vol. I, (Amos, B., ed.), Academic Press, New York and London, p. 35.

Milstein, C. P., Richardson, N. E., Deverson, E. V., and Feinstein, A. (1975). *Biochem. J.*, **151**, 615.

Montgomery, P. C., Dorrington, K. J., and Rockey, J. H. (1969). *Biochemistry*, **8**, 1427.

Morris, J. E., and Inman, F. P. (1968). *Biochemistry*, **7**, 2851.

Müller-Eberhard, H. J., and Kunkel, H. G. (1961). *Proc. Soc. Exp. Biol. Med.*, **106**, 291.

Natvig, J. B. (1966). *Nature (Lond.)*, **211**, 318.

Natvig, J. B., Gaarder, P. I., and Turner, M. W. (1972). *Clin. Exp. Immunol.*, **12**, 177.

Natvig, J. B., and Kunkel, H. G. (1973). *Adv. Immunol.*, **16**, 1.

Natvig, J. B., and Turner, M. W. (1970). *Nature (Lond.)*, **225**, 855.

Nisonoff, A., Hopper, J. E., and Spring, S. B. (1975). *The Antibody Molecule*, Academic Press, New York and London.

Normansell, D. E. (1970). *Immunochemistry*, **7**, 787.

Normansell, D. E. (1971). *Immunochemistry*, **8**, 593.

O'Donnell, I. J., Frangione, B., and Porter, R. R. (1970). *Biochem. J.*, **116**, 261.

Ogra, P. L., and Karzon, D. T. (1969). *J. Immunol.*, **102**, 15.

Okafor, G. O., and Turner, M. W. (1974). *Scand. J. Immunol.*, **3**, 181.

Okafor, G. O., Turner, M. W., and Hay, F. C. (1974). *Nature (Lond.)*, **248**, 228.

Oliveira, B., and Lamm, M. E. (1971). *Biochemistry*, **10**, 26.

Onoue, K., Kishimoto, T., and Yamamura, Y. (1968). *J. Immunol.*, **100**, 238.

Osterland, C. K., Harboe, M., and Kunkel, H. G. (1963). *Vox Sang*, **8**, 135.

Ovary, Z. (1960). *Immunology*, **3**, 19.

Ovary, Z., Barth, W. F., and Fahey, J. L. (1965). *J. Immunol.*, **94**, 410.

Parish, W. E. (1970). *J. Immunol.*, **105**, 1296.

Parish, W. E. (1974). In *Progress in Immunology II*, Vol. IV, (Brent, L., and Holborow, J., eds.), North Holland Publishing Co., Amsterdam, p. 19.

Parkhouse, R. M. E., Askonas, B. A., and Dourmashkin, R. R. (1970). *Immunology*, **18**, 575.

Pink, J. R., Buttery, S. H., De Vries, G. M., and Milstein, C. (1970). *Biochem. J.*, **117**, 33.

Plaut, A. G., and Tomasi, T. B., Jr. (1970). *Proc. Nat. Acad. Sci., U.S.A.*, **63**, 318.

Plaut, A. G., Wistar, R., and Capra, J. D. (1974). *J. Clin. Invest.*, **54**, 1295.

Poger, M. E., and Lamm, M. E. (1974). *J. Exp. Med.*, **139**, 629.

Poljak, R. J. (1975). *Nature (Lond.)*, **256**, 373.

Porter, R. R. (1959). *Biochem. J.*, **73**, 119.

Porter, R. R. (1962). *Symposium on Basic Problems in Neoplastic Disease* (Gelhorn, A., and Hirschberg, E., eds.), Columbia University Press, p. 177.

Putnam, F. W., Florent, G., Paul, C., Shinoda, T., and Shimizu, A. (1973a). *Science, N.Y.*, **182**, 287.

Putnam, F. W., Shinoda, T., Shimizu, A., Paul, C., Florent, G., and Raff, E. (1973b). In *3rd International Convocation on Immunology*, Kargel, Basel, p. 40.

Putnam, F. W., Titani, K., and Whitley, E. (1966). *Proc. Roy. Soc., Ser. B.*, **166**, 124.

Robboy, S. J., Lewis, E. J., Schur, P. H., and Colman, R. W. (1970). *Am. J. Med.*, **49**, 742.

Rose, H. M., Ragan, C., Pearce, E., and Lipman, M. O. (1948). *Proc. Soc. Exp. Biol. Med.*, **68**, 1.

Rowe, D. S., and Fahey, J. L. (1965a). *J. Exp. Med.*, **121**, 171.

Rowe, D. S., and Fahey, J. L. (1965b). *J. Exp. Med.*, **121**, 185.

Rowe, D. S., Hug, K., Forni, L., and Pernis, B. (1973). *J. Exp. Med.*, **138**, 965.

Saltvedt, E., and Harboe, M. (1976). *Scand. J. Immunol.*, **5**, 1103.

Sandberg, A. L., Oliveira, B., and Osler, A. G. (1971). *J. Immunol.*, **106**, 282.

56

Scholz, R., and Hilschmann, N. (1975). *Hoppe-Seyler's Z. Physiol. Chem.*, **356**, 1333.
Schur, P. H. (1972). In *Progress in Clinical Immunology*, Vol. I, (Schwartz, R., ed.), Grune and Stratton, New York, p. 71.
Segal, D. M., Padlan, E. A., Cohen, G. H., Silverton, E. W., Davies, D. R., Rudikoff, S., and Potter, M. (1974). In *Progress in Immunology II*, Vol. I, (Brent, L., and Holborow, J., eds.), North Holland Publishing Co., Amsterdam, p. 93.
Seon, B.-K., and Pressman, D. (1975). *Immunochemistry*, **12**, 333.
Sjöquist, J., and Stålenheim, G. (1969). *J. Immunol.*, **103**, 467.
Solheim, B. G., and Harboe, M. (1972). *Immunochemistry*, **9**, 623.
South, M. A., Cooper, M. D., Wolheim, F. A., Hong, R., and Good, R. A. (1966). *J. Exp. Med.*, **123**, 615.
Spiegelberg, H. L. (1974). *Adv. Immunol.*, **19**, 259.
Spiegelberg, H. L. (1975). *Nature (Lond.)*, **254**, 723.
Spiegelberg, H. L., and Götze, O. (1972). *Fed. Proc.*, **31**, 655.
Spiegelberg, H. L., Prahl, J. W., and Grey, H. M. (1970). *Biochemistry*, **9**, 2115.
Stålenheim, G., and Castensson, S. (1971). *FEBS Letters*, **14**, 79.
Stålenheim, G., and Malmheden-Eriksson, I. (1971). *FEBS Letters*, **14**, 82.
Stanworth, D. R. (1970). *Clin. Exp. Immunol.*, **6**, 1.
Stanworth, D. R. (1973). *Immediate Hypersensitivity*, North Holland Publishing Co., Amsterdam.
Stanworth, D. R., and Smith, A. K. (1973). *Clin. Allergy*, **3**, 37.
Stanworth, D. R., and Turner, M. W. (1973). In *Handbook of Experimental Immunology*, 2nd. Edition (Weir, D. M., ed.), Blackwell Scientific Publications, p. 10.1.
Steward, M. W., Turner, M. W., Natvig, J. B., and Gaarder, P. I. (1973). *Clin. Exp. Immunol.*, **15**, 145.
Strausbauch, P. H., Hurwitz, E., and Givol, D. (1971). *Biochemistry*, **10**, 2231.
Svasti, J., and Milstein, C. (1972). *Eur. J. Biochem.*, **31**, 405.

Terr, A. I., and Bentz, J. D. (1965). *J. Allergy*, **36**, 433.
Terry, W. D. (1966). *J. Immunol.*, **95**, 1041.
Terry, W. D., Fahey, J. L., and Steinberg, A. G. (1965). *J. Exp. Med.*, **122**, 1087.
Thompson, R. A. (1970). *Nature (Lond.)*, **226**, 946.
Tizard, I. R. (1969). *Int. Archs Allergy*, **36**, 332.
Turner, M. W. (1974). In *Progress in Immunology II*, Vol. I, (Brent, L., and Holborow, J., eds.), North Holland Publishing Co., Amsterdam, p. 280.
Turner, M. W., and Bennich, H. (1968). *Biochem. J.*, **107**, 71.
Turner, M. W., Bennich, H., and Natvig, J. B. (1970). *Clin. Exp. Immunol.*, **7**, 603.
Turner, M. W., Komvopoulos, A., Bennich, H., and Natvig, J. B. (1972). *Scand. J. Immunol.*, **1**, 53.
Turner, M. W., Mårtensson, L., Natvig, J. B., and Bennich, H. (1969). *Nature (Lond.)*, **221**, 1166.

Vaerman, J. P., and Heremans, J. F. (1966). *Science, N.Y.*, **153**, 647.
Valentine, R. C., and Green, N. M. (1967). *J. Mol. Biol.*, **27**, 615.
van der Giessen, M. (1975). Doctoral thesis, University of Amsterdam.
Virella, G., Nunes, M. A-S., and Tamagnini, G. (1972). *Clin. Exp. Immunol.*, **10**, 475.

Waaler, E. (1940). *Acta path. microbiol. scand.*, **17**, 172.
Waldmann, T. A., and Hemmings, W. A. (1974). In *Progress in Immunology II*, Vol. I, (Brent, L., and Holborow, J., eds.), North Holland Publishing Co., Amsterdam, p. 230.
Waldmann, T. A., and Strober, W. (1969). *Prog. Allergy*, **13**, 1.
Waldmann, T. A., Strober, W., and Blaese, R. M. (1971). In *Progress in Immunology*, Vol. I, (Amos, B., ed.), Academic Press, New York, p. 891.

Waller, M., and Vaughan, J. H. (1956). *Proc. Soc. Exp. Biol. Med.*, **92**, 198.

Wang, A. C., Faulk, W. P., Stukey, A. M. A., and Fudenberg, H. H. (1970). *Immunochemistry*, **7**, 703.

Wang, A. C., van Loghem, E., and Shuster, J. (1973). *Fed. Proc.*, **32**, 1003.

Watanabe, S., Barnikol, H. U., Horn, J., Bertram, J., and Hilschmann, N. (1973). *Hoppe Seyler's Z. Physiol. Chem.*, **354**, 1505.

Watkins, J., Turner, M. W., and Roberts, A. (1971). In *Protides of the Biological Fluids*, (Peeters, H., ed.), Pergamon Press, Oxford and New York, p. 461.

Wells, J. V., Bleumers, J. F., and Fudenberg, H. H. (1973). *Proc. Nat. Acad. Sci. U.S.A.*, **70**, 827.

Welscher, H. D. (1970). *Nature (Lond.)*, **228**, 1236.

Wolfenstein-Todel, C., Prelli, F., Frangione, B., and Franklin, E. C. (1973). *Biochemistry*, **12**, 5195.

Wu, T. T., and Kabat, E. A. (1970). *J. Exp. Med.*, **132**, 211.

Wolfenstein-Todel, C., Frangione, B., Prelli, F., and Franklin, E. C. (1976). *Biochemical and Biophysical Research Communications*, **71**, 907.

Yasmeen, D., Ellerson, J. R., Dorrington, K. J., and Painter, R. H. (1973). *J. Immunol.*, **110**, 1706.

Yount, W. J., Dorner, M. M., Kunkel, H. G., and Kabat, E. A. (1968). *J. Exp. Med.*, **127**, 633.

CHAPTER 2

Antigen-Combining Region of Immunoglobulins

F. F. Richards, J. M. Varga,
R. W. Rosenstein, and W. H. Konigsberg

1 ANTIBODY COMBINING REGION STRUCTURE

1.1 Combining Region Specificity

Stimulation by antigen evokes the production of immunoglobulins in the serum and secretions of vertebrates. A common property of these induced proteins is the ability to bind antigen. The ligating function of the immunoglobulin molecule is predominantly the property of the combining regions, which are two symmetrical areas at the solvent-exposed ends of the Fab arms of the Y-shaped immunoglobulin molecules. The combining region is situated in the variable (V region) domain, a compact region consisting of the N-terminal half of the light chain and the N-terminal quarter of the heavy chain which are linked by sulphydryl bonds. Between the areas of this domain occupied by the light and heavy chain variable regions is a cleft exposed to the solvent, in or close to which antigens have been shown to bind (Amzel *et al.*, 1974). An induced antibody population is said to be specific because it usually binds most strongly to the immunizing antigen and less strongly to other compounds which structurally resemble the immunogen. Occasionally, antibodies (heteroclitic) are induced which bind more strongly to some determinant other than the immunogen (Mäkelä *et al.*, 1975). In general, antibody populations show a high degree of specificity in that they are able to discriminate between chemical compounds differing by as little as a single functional group, between stereoisomers, or between two proteins differing by as little as a single amino acid residue (Reichlin, 1974, Richards *et al.*, 1975).

The number of individual immunoglobulins in an immune serum may be quite large. It is not unusual to see as many as 50 protein bands on isoelectric focusing, all of which are capable of binding the immunogen, but such a population of immunoglobulins does not behave uniformly with respect to ligand binding. In fact, subpopulations can be identified that bind ligand over a wide range of intrinsic binding constants (K_A) (Eisen, 1964a, Eisen and Siskind, 1964). This, in turn, suggests that the antigen combining sites also show corresponding variations of structure. This structural heterogeneity is further complicated by a degree of temporal heterogeneity, since during the immune response the composition of the antibody population does not remain constant (Steiner and Eisen, 1966; Steiner and Eisen, 1967*a*, *b*; Steward and Petty, 1972; Macario and Conway de Macario, 1975). New antibodies appear while others disappear, suggesting that the antibodies expressed at any one time during the immune response are only a small proportion of the total number with complementarity to the immunizing antigen that the animal is capable of producing. Thus, the immune response is very heterogeneous but, when viewed as a population, also highly specific with respect to antigen binding. This chapter will explore the structural basis of antibody specificity.

1.2 General Properties of Combining Regions

The first quantitative assessments of the number of antigen molecules and antibody molecules in antigen–antibody complexes suggested that 7 S antibody molecules are bivalent (Porter and Press, 1962). This conclusion was reinforced by ultracentrifugal studies (Nisonoff and Thorbecke, 1964), and when accurate values for the molecular weights of antibody molecules became available, the dimeric nature of the binding units (Cohen and Porter, 1964) confirmed this hypothesis.

Both heavy and light chains are necessary for optimal binding. Experiments that tested isolated light or heavy chains for their ability to ligate hapten showed that isolated light chains have little ability to bind, although with sensitive methods low-affinity binding of haptens can be detected (Yoo *et al.*, 1967; Painter *et al.*, 1972). Isolated heavy chains are generally insoluble, but when rendered soluble one mole of heavy chain generally binds one mole of antigen. However, the binding affinity of isolated heavy chains is greatly reduced (Utsumi and Karush, 1964), even though the ability to discriminate between related antigens is retained (Haber and Richards, 1967).

Experiments in Porter's laboratory showed that papain digestion of the IgG molecule produces Fab fragments containing the whole light chain and the N-terminal half of the heavy chain. These Fab fragments were shown to bind antigen with a valence of one (Porter, 1958). Pepsin digestion of some myeloma immunoglobulins under controlled conditions gives a fragment which consists of the N-terminal half—or in the nomenclature of Konigsberg and of Edelman, the first domain (Waxdal *et al.*, 1968; Edelman *et al.*, 1969)—of the Fab fragment (Inbar *et al.*, 1972). This fragment (Fv) contains the variable N-terminal half of the light chain and the N-terminal variable quarter of the heavy chain. The Fv fragment retains the binding function of the Fab fragment and carries the idiotypic (or combining region-related) antigenic determinants of the immunoglobulin molecule (Figure 1). Such studies show that the 7 S unit of immunoglobulins has two combining regions located at the N-terminal ends of the Fab fragments and that both the light and heavy chains are necessary for maximal antigen binding.

On the basis of fluorescence polarization studies, Edelman originally proposed that the combining regions were situated at either end of a long, rod-like molecule (Weltman and Edelman, 1967), but the electron micrographs of Feinstein and Rowe (1965), followed by the detailed pictures of bivalent hapten–antigen complexes by Valentine and Green (1967) and by Green, (1969) left little doubt that the molecule is in fact Y-shaped, with the combining regions occupying the ends of the two Fab arms. In addition, the experiments by Valentine and Green

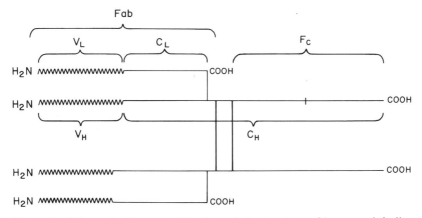

Figure 1 Schematic diagram of the four-chain structure of immunoglobulin. V_L and V_H are the variable regions of the light and heavy chains; C_L and C_H are the constant regions. The antigen-binding sites, one each heavy–light chain pair, are made up of amino acid residues from the variable regions. Fab and Fc are the fragments produced by papain digestion of immunoglobulin

(1967) showed that the site binding the dinitrophenyl hapten (DNP) is some distance below the surface of the molecule, since bivalent DNP antigens, in which the two DNP groups are connected by a short spacer moiety, fail to form head-to-head immunoglobulin polymers. This supports earlier observations indicating a hydrophobic environment for the DNP-binding site, thus suggesting that the site is located below the surface (Little and Eisen, 1967). Other experiments have indicated that the Fab arms are movable with respect to each other and the Fc fragment (Yguerabide *et al.*, 1970; Cathou *et al.*, 1974).

Thus, prior to X-ray crystallographic analysis, a speculative picture had emerged of a combining region located at the ends of the movable Fab arms, containing a cleft or cavity, surrounded by both light and heavy chain variable regions. It is remarkable how accurately the antigen-probe methods were able to predict the probable size and shape of the combining region which have been substantiated by X-ray crystallography.

1.3 Immunological Probes for Combining Regions

The antibody molecule itself is antigenic both when injected into heterologous species (Brient *et al.*, 1971) and when introduced into mice of the same inbred strain from which the immunizing antibody is derived (Sirisinha and Eisen, 1971). In heterologous immunization, the quantitatively dominant immunogenic region is the Fc fragment of the molecule. For instance, an anti-rabbit serum of sheep has most of its binding activity directed against rabbit Fc regions. When homogeneous immunoglobulins are introduced into a homologous inbred mouse line—when a mouse myeloma tumour immunoglobulin derived from a BALB/c mouse is injected repeatedly into other BALB/c mice—levels of antibodies to the Fc region are relatively low in titre and antibodies appear which react with Fab fragments. These antibodies were believed to recognize only the inducing myeloma protein and were therefore called anti-idiotypic (Nisonoff *et al.*, 1975). A characteristic of a proportion of the early anti-idiotype sera is that the idiotype–anti-idiotype interaction is inhibited to some extent by antigen (Brient *et al.*, 1971). The Fv region of a mouse myeloma (derived from tumour MOPC 315) is able to adsorb the anti-idiotypic activity of a mouse serum induced by immunization with protein 315, and that it therefore contains all the idiotypic determinants (Haimovich *et al.*, 1972). The Fv fragments has previously been shown to contain one V region of the light chain and the whole V region. Comparative sequential analysis by Wu and Kabat (1970), and by Capra and Kehoe, (1976) identified three groups of amino acid residues within the V_L and V_H regions which are more variable than other residues in this region. These hypervariable residues were shown by X-ray diffraction analysis to be located on the outside of six polypeptide loops on the free distal region of the N-terminal domain which are accessible to solvent and which surround the antibody combining region (Padlan *et al.*, 1974; Poljak *et al.*, 1974). Isolated light and heavy chains are capable of inhibiting the idiotype–anti-idiotype interaction (Hoessli *et al.*, 1976). From these data, it seems reasonable to deduce that anti-idiotypic sera are directed against the solvent-accessible regions and hypervariable loops of the N-terminal domain. Since whole light chains may be common to two different antibodies and since sequential data suggest that whole hypervariable loops may have structures that resemble each other, anti-idiotypic sera are clearly not anti-idiotypic in the sense that they can characterize only one combining region.

The lack of idiotypy in these determinants also has been recognized experimentally. The literature abounds in terms such as 'shared idiotypic specificities' which have been recognized not only between different mouse strains (Kuettner et al., 1972), but also between different species (Varga et al., 1974). Anti-idiotype antibodies, therefore, are not antibodies which define a unique set on V-region structures. In this chapter the term antibodies to V regions will henceforth be used.

The relationship between the antigen-binding capacity of a single V region and the antibodies raised against the V region has been studied in detail (Potter and Lieberman, 1970; Lieberman et al., 1975). It is concluded that antibodies may be prepared complementary to a region of a myeloma protein binding a determinant such as phosphorylcholine. These antibodies cross-react with some, but generally not with all, myeloma V regions binding the same antigenic determinant. Those myeloma proteins which cross-react with the same anti-V-region serum generally show the same fine specificity, that is, they all bind a series of haptens related to the antigenic determinant. Thus, it appears that there may be several families of antibodies complementary to a single antigen and that such families may be distinguished from each other by anti-V-region sera. Similar considerations apply also to antibodies elicited by antigens (Lieberman et al., 1974).

Antibodies to V regions are inhibited by antigens to different extents, and this can be understood if it is remembered that bound antigens may encroach on different solvent-exposed loops to varying degrees, and that anti-V-region sera are not necessarily directed against all loops to the same degree. An interesting method has been developed by Claflin and his associates (Claflin and Davie, 1975) in which antibodies to V regions are bound to affinity columns containing the requisite V regions attached to the solid support. The bound antibodies are eluted with haptens, thus displacing only those immunoglobulins that are directed against loops in close apposition to the hapten-binding site. By exploiting the multiple binding potential of a single binding region, it should be possible to produce serological probes directed against individual peptides within the combining region, a potentially useful tool for probing the structure of the combining region.

Since antibodies to V regions may bind in the same general area as antigens, they appear to be able to mimic some of the physiological consequences of antigen binding and to induce a limited immune response (Cosenza and Kohler, 1972). Also, they can blanket the combining region, preventing the antigen gaining access, thereby inhibiting the immune response. For this reason, control or suppression of certain antibodies by anti-V-region antibodies has been considered recently. The bimodal nature of the reaction of antibodies to V regions has suggested to some workers that antibodies to the second, third, or perhaps even higher degree may form a network controlling the immune response (Jerne, 1974). Whether or not this theoretical web is anchored firmly remains to be determined. Among the more recent practical uses of anti-V-region antibodies has been an attempt to investigate the nature of antigen-binding receptors on T lymphocytes. The results of these experiments have suggested that V-region antigens are present on, or close to, the antigen-recognition site of T lymphocytes (Binz *et al.*, 1974). This suggests that a recognition mechanism, which has some common features with immunoglobulin V regions, is also present on the T cells. This area is at present under investigation.

1.4 Polymeric Ligand Probes

An important method, which accurately predicted the size of the combining region, was devised originally by Kabat (1960). If there is point-to-point contact with antigen in the antibody combining region, one should be able to raise antibodies to homopolymers of the type $(X-X-X)_n$, where n is a large number. Monomers, dimers, trimers, tetramers, and oligomers of X may be prepared and their ability to inhibit the reaction between the X polymer and the antibody may be determined. It was reasoned that, on a molar basis, the inhibition of the oligomers should increase until the combining region is filled completely, and after this, increasing the size of competing molecule should have no further effect on the inhibition. In his original experiments, Kabat used dextran for immunization and found that polysaccharides containing up to five or six glucose units inhibited maximally and that thereafter, increasing length did not have any further effect on inhibition. From these data he suggested that the combining region could be as large as $3\cdot4 \times 1\cdot2 \times 0\cdot7$ nm, the extended measurement of the isomaltohexaose unit. Kabat also noted that there was evidence of heterogeneity in the type of contact which was made. Using some sera, the isomaltotroise unit is almost as efficient an inhibitor as the isomaltohexaose (Kabat, 1960).

Numerous laboratories have repeated these experiments using other homopolymers, such as polypeptides and polynucleotides, as well as random amino acid copolymers. The conclusions of these studies are that the size of the site is compatible with binding extended polymers of the size range $2\cdot5-3\cdot6 \times 1\cdot0-1\cdot7 \times 0\cdot6-0\cdot7$ nm. More recently, careful quantitative studies using polyalanine (Schechter *et al.*, 1970) and using antibodies to blood group A substance, inhibited by various polysaccharides (Moreno and Kabat, 1969), have substantiated that the binding energy is incremental with each added unit and that antibody–antigen contact in these complexes must extend over a relatively large area.

Similar methods have been used to determine if there is any variation in the average size of the combining region during the changes in antibody population that occur during maturation of the immune response, using polyasparagine was used as antigen. It was concluded that there is some increase in average site dimensions during maturation (Murphy and Sage, 1970).

1.5 Affinity and Photoaffinity Probes

A chemically reactive ligand, which initially is bound by non-covalent interactions at the binding site of a ligating protein, can be induced to react with the protein, resulting in the formation of covalent bonds. If these bonds are sufficiently stable, the protein may be digested chemically or enzymatically into peptides and the location in the primary sequence of the amino acid residues modified by the affinity reagent determined. This method used in enzymology was introduced into immunology by Wofsy *et al.* (1962) and has been used extensively to study the combining regions of both myeloma proteins and whole antibody populations directed against antigenic determinants (Singer and Doolittle, 1966; Knowles, 1972; Givol, 1974).

Affinity reagents consist of chemically reactive moieties which are attached to, or are an integral part of, a haptenic determinant. Such reagents depend entirely on the higher concentrations of the reagents at, or near, the combining region for differential labelling. No evidence of special reactivity of a single amino acid side chain within the immunoglobulin combining region is available. Since concentration differences are a crucial factor in affinity labelling, high affinity of the immunoglobulin for the hapten and a low molar ratio of ligand to immunoglobulin combining region will favour site-related labelling. At higher ligand levels, local accumulations of ligand in regions of the protein not related to the high-affinity site are likely to increase and may modify the protein in these regions. Protection of the combining region by the hapten itself is used as an index of site-directed labelling. However, when there is a considerable difference in K_A between hapten and the hapten-based affinity reagents, the possibility of nonequivalence of the two binding processes should be considered.

In practice, only two types of reactive groups have been used as affinity reagents with immunoglobulins. Wofsy *et al.* (1962) used diazonium fluoroborate to label antibody-combining regions. These fluoroborates are relatively stable salts, which react with amino groups of proteins, the ε-amino groups of lysine, and the phenol ring of tyrosine; reaction of this diazonium salt with histidine has also been reported (Wofsy and Parker, 1967). The stability and ease of synthesis recommend this reagent. However, the limited reactivity may mean that the contact site itself may not be labelled, but rather that reaction occurs at the nearest or most reactive tyrosine, lysine, or histidine residue. The haloketone compounds employed as affinity reagents by Givol, Eisen and their associates (Haimovich *et al.*, 1970; Eisen, 1971; Haimovich *et al.*, 1972; Givol, 1974) have similar strengths and weaknesses. Their spectrum of reactivity with amino acids resembles that of the diazonium salts. Since all affinity reagents are introduced into the aqueous solvent and enter the combining site by diffusion, the rate of hydrolysis of such reagents must be slow, thus limiting both the spectrum of reactivity and the concentrations in which the reagent may be used.

If a non-reactive labelling reagent could be placed at the combining site, and if within the combining site the non-reactive labelling reagent could be activated to produce a moiety capable of forming covalent bonds with the antibody protein then some, but by no means all, of the difficulties associated with affinity reagents might be ameliorated. Converse and Richards (1968; 1969) synthesized a DNP-based diazoketone of the type described earlier by Vaughan and Westheimer (1969), which may be photoactivated to a carbene or a ketene, the former authors showed that this reagent with anti-DNP antibodies. Fleet *et al.* (1969) introduced another light-activated compound, an aromatic azide, for the same purpose (Fisher and Press, 1974).

It is possible to isolate antibody–reagent complexes and to activate these specifically, although for this a relatively high binding energy for the hapten–antibody complex is needed. However, the major advantage is that some molecules of these reagents are in contact with the protein very shortly after they are generated and do not first pass through the solvent. Most reagents that are highly reactive with protein will also react with aqueous solvents. By generating highly reactive reagents *in situ*, it is possible to label specifically residue side chains. For instance, the activated carbenes are potentially capable of inserting into any carbon–heteroatomic linkage, and it is probable that the nitrenes generated by light from the aromatic azido compounds have a similar broad range of reactivity. It must be remembered, however, that light will activate not only those molecules of labelling reagent immobilized at the site, but also those in the vicinity of the site. Moreover, if the half life of the activated species is sufficiently long, migration of the activated species may occur (Hew *et al.*, 1973; Yoshioka *et al.*, 1973; Lifter *et al.*, 1974; Richards *et al.*, 1974). It has been suggested that scavenger molecule should be employed to deal with the wandering activated photoaffinity label molecules (Ruoho *et al.*, 1973). However, such molecules may react with the activated reagent bound at the site, and since scavenger molecules may themselves form low-affinity interactions with the protein, there is a possibility at least that an already complex system will become even more complicated due to such corrective measures. A second approach has been to synthesize photoaffinity reagents with shorter chemical half lives, such as the azulene reagents (Smith and Knowles, 1973).

The chemistry of affinity and photoaffinity reagents has been introduced in some detail since it is difficult to interpret results of the exploration of antibody combining regions without adequate knowledge. Although it is probable that no single reagent is ideal, it is hoped that a consensus of the labelling information will provide some understanding of the binding properties of immunoglobulins. However, no easy general conclusions are possible: but in general, modifications occur at, or near, some of the hypervariable regions. There are, however, two reports of labelling outside the accepted hypervariable regions (Franek, 1973; Richards *et al.*, 1974); some residues, such as the tyrosine at position 33 or 34 in the light chain, are modified in a number of different experiments. There is, reasonable doubt that this is a contact amino acid residue, as it is a constant residue within a hypervariable region. Modification of this residue reduces the strength of binding, but does not affect the number of DNP groups which can be bound (Goetzl and Metzger, 1970). The same residue is modified both by nitrophenol affinity reagents in anti-DNP immunoglobulins and by a phosphorylcholine-based reagent in a phosphorylcholine-binding myeloma protein. Also, in labelling experiments on myeloma protein 460, the modified residues may well be so far apart as to make it unlikely that these residues can have been modified by a reagent binding to only a single site within each Fab fragment.

To summarize, it seems likely that affinity reagents do modify amino acid residues in the general combining region. It may be that, in some instances, they modify contact amino acids of a single major binding site. In other cases, a number of different binding sites (perhaps with a wide range of binding affinities) is modified. There is no *a priori* reason why only one high-affinity binding site should be modified (Richards *et al.*, 1974) if others of lower affinity are also present (Haselkorn *et al.*, 1974). While the original expectations of affinity labelling may have been unduly simple, affinity and photoaffinity labelling methods may still be valuable tools for studying the complex geometry of hapten ligation to antibodies.

1.6 Physicochemical Probes of Antibody Combining Regions

The properties of all molecules are affected by their environment. With certain molecules, changes in property between the molecule in solution and the molecule bound to an immunoglobulin combining region may be observed directly. The observed effects of physical and chemical alterations on binding may include differences in ionization (Albertson and Phillipson, 1960), solubility properties (Day *et al.*, 1963), and increases or decreases in fluorescence either of the protein or of the ligand in the rotatory dispersion of light, in the circular dichroism of polarized light, and in the circular dichroism of polarized emitted fluorescent light (Schlessinger *et al.*, 1975). The magnetic properties, as well as the electron spin resonance of ligand and ligating molecule, also may be affected by binding (Dwek *et al.*, 1975a). Sensitive calorimetric methods can measure changes in enthalpy, and indirectly, changes in the entropy during antibody–antigen interaction can be determined (Johnston *et al.*, 1974). Variations in the rotatory behaviour of whole immunoglobulin molecules on binding large antigens can be monitored by the depolarization of emitted fluorescence; even changes in specific molar volume have been observed (Ohta *et al.*, 1970). More recently, the internal patterns of movement of macromolecules (the concerted breaking and reforming of hydrogen bonds which have been described as the 'breathing' of the molecule and which may affect ligand binding) have been observed. This wealth of physicochemical information is discussed by Feinstein and Beale in Chapter 8 of this volume and in other review articles (Day, 1972; Cathou *et al.*, 1974).

It is perhaps disappointing how little direct information this work on combining-region structure and function has yielded in comparison to X-ray diffraction analysis. It seems likely that as with other proteins, the largest and most important contributions these methods may have to make is yet to come. It is in the fine analysis of mechanism of macromolecules whose overall anatomy is understood that these methods are most useful.

The areas in which physicochemical probes have given the most information about the combining region have been the depth and hydrophobicity of the combining sites, the involvement of light and heavy chains in ligand binding, and the unexpected degree to which small ligands stabilize the light–heavy chain interaction. Physicochemical methods also have been a mainstay in the assessment of possible conformational changes secondary to antigen binding.

X-ray crystallographic studies quoted in Section 1.8 show that in the two antibody V regions so far examined both the small ligand (phosphorylcholine) and a larger one (γ-hydroxy vitamin K_1) appear to make contact with both the light and heavy chains. Nevertheless, the area of contact of phosphorycholine with the light chain is small. It is known, however, that light–heavy chain contacts in the V and C_1 domains of the Fab fragment are extensive and involve many amino acid residues. It is, therefore, somewhat surprising that small ligands such as the DNP moiety can stabilize light–heavy chain interaction to a considerable degree. Light and heavy chains may be isolated from reduced and alkylated IgG in dissociating solvents by gel filtration. Metzger and Singer (1963) found that light and heavy chain yields are reduced considerably when the small DNP antigen is present in the mixture. Optical rotatory dispersion studies by Cathou and Haber (1967) and by Cathou and Werner (1970) showed also that the presence of the DNP hapten greatly reduces the unfolding of antibody molecules in the dissociating agent, quanidine hydrochloride. Thus, antibody without the DNP ligand unfolds in the presence of guanidine hydrochloride (2 N), while in the presence of the ligand, binding activity is still intact in the presence of a higher concentration of guanidine hydrochloride (4 N). Yet isolated heavy chains derived from DNP antibodies still show binding activity, albeit with a greatly reduced K_A, which may be due to the presence of new structures resembling the combining regions formed from heavy-chain dimers (Stevenson, 1973).

When tryptophan is excited by ultraviolet light at 280 nm, it fluoresces at 345 nm. Tryptophan residues are found in close association with the combining region. Introduction of a DNP or a folic acid group into the combining region will absorb emitted tryptophan fluorescence usually. The quenching of fluorescence has been used both as a structural tool and as an indication of hapten binding. The wavelength of maximal absorption of incident light exhibited by ligands such as DNP also may be red-shifted by binding to the protein (Eisen, 1964b). The observed spectral changes have suggested to some workers that charge–transfer complexes may be formed between aromatic ligands and residues such as tryptophan. However, convincing evidence for the presence of charge–transfer complexes remains elusive (Rubinstein and Little, 1970). It is now well recognized that a large number of different V regions may bind small ligands such as DNP with K_0 ranging from 10^{-11} to 10^{-4} M. It is unlikely that such a wide range of binding energies can be consistent with one type of DNP-binding site.

Optical spectrophotometric evidence for conformational changes secondary to antigen binding has been dealt with elsewhere (see Schlessinger *et al.*, 1975. The introduction of electron spin resonance probes (Stryer and Griffith, 1965; Hsia and Piette, 1969; Piette *et al.*, 1972) has added an additional tool for the study of combining regions. These workers used haptens which had been linked previously to moieties containing the nitroxide spin label. When the hapten is firmly fixed to the nitroxide spin label, it can be shown that the complex is firmly bound. By producing molecules in which the hapten and the spin label are separated by chemical spacer groups of various lengths, the degree of rotational freedom of the spin label can be estimated as a function of spacer length. Some information on the size or depth of the combining region can be extrapolated from this information.

The lanthanide element series bind both to the Fc and Fv region of antibody molecules. In rabbit IgG, the Fc binding constant is around 5×10^{-6} M, while those in the combining region have a K_0 of around 10^{-4} M for gadolinum. It has been shown that, in a DNP-binding IgA myeloma protein, the gadolinum (Gd III)-binding site is close to that of DNP and that the binding of DNP weakens the attachment of lanthanide (Dower *et al.*, 1975; Dwek *et al.*, 1975b). The same workers have shown also by using Piette's technique that the portion of the combining region binding DNP probably measures $1 \cdot 1 \times 0 \cdot 9 \times 0 \cdot 6$ nm, based on nitroxide spin labels. Proton nuclear magnetic resonance spectroscopy at 270 MH gives a paramagnetic difference spectrum, which suggests that about 30 aliphatic and 30 aromatic residues are involved around the DNP-combining site.

1.7 Electron Microscopic Probes

Although early biophysical studies had suggested that the viscosity of the IgG molecule was consistent with the interpretation that was composed of three independently moving units with molecular weights of approximately 50 000 (Noellsen *et al.*, 1965), the first convincing demonstration that it is, in fact, Y-shaped and that the two combining regions are located at the ends of the two movable arms of the Y, came from electron microscopy. The studies of Lafferty and Oertelis (1963) and of Almeida and Waterson (1969) showed viruses with thread-like structures which formed U-shaped bands on the viral surface, while Feinstein and Rowe (1965) demonstrated ferritin molecules held together by thin, angled molecules. Valentine and Green (1967) used bifunctional DNP haptens which were separated from each by carbon skeletons of various lengths. With the bifunctional antigen containing an eight-carbon skeleton, DNP–NH–$(CH_2)_8$–NH–DNP, excellent cross-linked complexes were obtained in which the combining region of one molecule was joined head-to-head with the combining region of the next molecule (Figure 2). The electron microscopic field at a magnification of $\times 400\ 000$ shows predominantly ring-shaped structures of various sizes with knobs protruding outwards. These rings are composed of two, three, four, or more molecules of IgG joined by their combining regions and held together by the bifunctional antigen. The knob can be removed with pepsin, an enzyme known to cleave the Fc fragment from the dimeric F(ab)$_2$ fragment. When bifunctional DNP antigens with a carbon skeleton of five or less were tested with protein 315, an anti-DNP mouse IgA myeloma protein, no ring structures were produced.

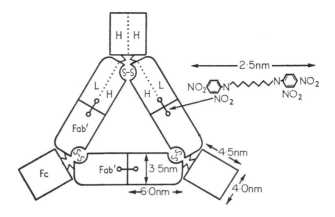

Figure 2 Diagrammatic representation of complexes of anti-DNP–IgG with bivalent DNP ligands. The electron micrographs on which this diagram is based gave the major dimensions of the IgG molecule, and the locations of the combining regions and the Fc fragment. The electron micrographs also demonstrated the flexibility of the Fab region at the hinge region of the molecule. By courtesy of Dr. N. M. Green and the Journal of Molecular Biology

These dramatic electron micrographs show (*i*) that the IgG and IgA molecules are Y-shaped, and (*ii*) that the arms are movable about a hinge-like region. Unlike previous studies, deformation of the molecule due to fixation on the carbon grid cannot be invoked to explain the different angles which Fab segments exhibited with respect to each other. The circular structures had clearly closed prior to fixation on the grid, demonstrating that flexibility of the Fab fragments with respect to each other is a functional feature of the molecule. The failure to form circular structures with short bifunctional haptens suggests that the DNP-binding site is at least 1·5 nm below the surface of the protein and that a cleft or cavity is probably present at the free end of the Fab fragment (Green, 1969). The major dimensions of the molecule can be measured from the electron micrographs. The Fab fragment containing the combining region has been estimated as 6·0 nm long and 3·5 nm broad. Careful examination of the IgA protein 315 molecules and of the IgG molecules showed that each Fab region is composed of two compact, round structures, giving visual evidence of the immunoglobulin sulphydryl-linked molecule domains which had been proposed on structural grounds by Edelman, Konigsberg, and their collaborators (Waxdal *et al.*, 1968). More recently, electron micrographs of a human IgG1 myeloma protein crystal using an optical averaging method have confirmed the Y-shaped structure of the whole molecule and the dimensions of the Fab fragment (Labow and Davies, 1971).

1.8 X-Ray Crystallography of Combining Regions

Northrop (1942) described the first crystalline preparation derived from trypsin-treated antibody and a number of investigators subsequently reported crystalline antibodies or antibody fragments (see, for example, Nisonoff *et al.*, 1967; *Hochman et al.*, 1973). The first Fab fragment crystals, however, which had potential for high resolution X-ray analysis only became available in the late 1960s. A human IgG1 myeloma, protein NEW, was analysed at 0·2 nm resolution by Poljak *et al.* (1974) and a mouse IgA myeloma protein derived from the McPc 603 tumour was studied by Segal *et al.* (1974) at a resolution of 0·2 nm. A third myeloma protein has been studied extensively by Edmundson, Schiffer, and their collaborators (Schiffer *et al.*, 1973; Edmundson *et al.*, 1974); this is a λ light-chain dimer associated with the McG human myeloma protein. In addition, Fehlhammer *et al.* (1975) and Epp *et al.* (1975) have compared the structure at 0·2 nm resolution of two κ light-chain dimers, Au and Rei, which differ in structure by only 16 amino acid residues.

At the time of writing, detailed information is available about the antigen-combining region complex of one human IgG myeloma (NEW), one mouse γA combining region–antigen complex (McPc 603), and three light-chain dimer models of the combining region (from Mcg, Au, and Rei).

Knowledge of the three-dimensional structure of the combining region has answered or potentially can answer a number of questions about antibody specificity. (*i*) What is the extent of the region complementary to antigen? (*ii*) Can several diverse antigen-binding sites be demonstrated in the combining region? (*iii*) The V region has a common folding pattern associated with areas of conserved amino acid sequence, in spite of which, it shows very large variation of antigen-binding specificity. By what mechanism is structural variation in binding sites created? (*iv*) Why is antigen binding predominantly to the combining region? What physical characteristics found in this region only, facilitate binding? (*v*) What are the structural consequences of antigen ligation? Are physiologically important conformational changes found secondary to antigen binding? If so, are these conformational signals transmitted to the Fc region or does some other mechanism occur?

A comparison of the structure of the variable domain shows some striking similarities between proteins NEW and McPc 603 (Poljak, 1975). Firstly, the basic immunoglobulin fold of the V-region polypeptides is essentially the same in both proteins, the same fold being found in the V_L and the V_H regions. The only difference is that the second light-chain hypervariable region is absent from NEW and the polypeptide backbone bridges across the base of the loop. A single disulphide bond links cysteine residues at loci equivalent to positions 26 and 85 on the light chain. The polypeptide backbone is principally in parallel folds in the form of β-pleated sheets, and there are no substantial α-helical segments. There are two sets of loops at either end of the V region of each chain (see Figures 3 and 4). One set of loops makes contact with the first constant domain; the other set are free in the sense that they are exposed to solvent. These three solvent-exposed

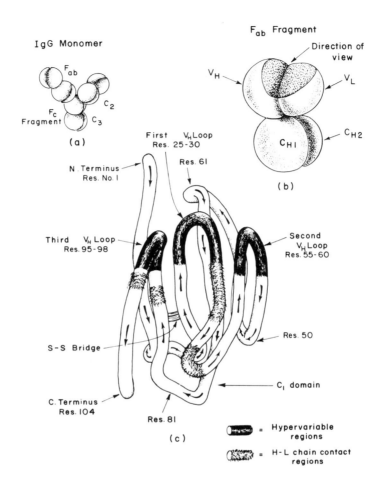

Figure 3 (*a*) The arrangement of the six domains of the antibody molecule with respect to each other. (*b*) An exploded diagram of the variable domain showing the V_L–V_H contact surface. (*c*) The polypeptide backbone fold of the heavy chain indicating the areas in contact with the light chain and the approximate location of the hypervariable regions. Redrawn from data on the NEW immunoglobulin molecule from Poljak *et al.* (1973) and Poljak (1975)

loops correspond approximately to the hypervariable regions. Hypervariable regions centre on residues 25–30, 50, and 95–100 of the light chain and residues 30, 55–60, and 105–110 of the heavy chain. It must be remembered that these are not rigidly bounded areas, the extent of hypervariability will depend on whether all light chains, κ or λ, or chains within each κ or λ subgroups are compared. The greater the difference between the groups and subgroups, the more extensive the region of hypervariability. While hypervariable residues in mouse and man occur in the area of the combining region there is no evidence to suggest that these are

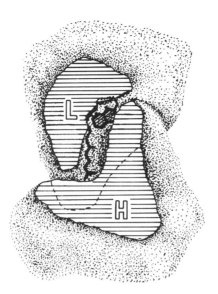

Figure 4 Scheme of the combining region of protein NEW looking into the long axis of the Fab fragment. The areas labelled L and H are occupied by the light and heavy chain, respectively. Between lies a depression approximately 0·5–0·6 nm deep in which the γ-hydroxy of vitamin K_1 molecule is located

obligatory contact residues for antigens. The X-ray evidence indicates that some hypervariable residues are in contact with antigen, while others are close and still more do not make contact. Contact is also made by antigen with regions other than the hypervariable ones (Poljak, 1975). In the rabbit, the relationship between hypervariability and antigen contact is even less certain (Haber *et al.*, 1975). It is probable that hypervariability does not reflect only the variation in amino acid sequence needed to bind directly to antigen. Compensatory sequence changes in regions away from the contact residues may also give rise to hypervariability. The predictions made from analysis of variability have proved very valuable in showing the general area in which antigen binding takes place.

In other regions of the back-bone polypeptide fold, the side chains of residues are involved in heavy–light chain interactions. These include residues 35, 37, 42, 43, 86, and 99 in the V_L and C_L, and residues 37, 39, 43, 45, 47, 95, and 108 in the V_H region of protein NEW (Poljak, 1975). These interacting residues are mainly, although not exclusively, hydrophobic and their presence does not appear to correlate with the heavy or light chain subgroup or light chain class, suggesting that there is no rigid restriction on the recombination of heavy and light chains. The V_L and V_H regions are essentially similar in shape. On association, they interact to form a roughly spherical domain, with the solvent-exposed distal end forming an approximately flat plate fringed by the hypervariable loops. Between the areas occupied by the light and heavy chains on this plate runs a cleft which is approximately 1·5–1·7 nm long. In the protein NEW, this cleft is shallow (Figure 5), perhaps 0·5–0·6 nm deep, while in protein 603 it is 1·2 nm deep, 1·5 nm wide, and 2·0 nm long (Poljak *et al.*, 1974). The light chain of protein 603 is of the κ type and has an insertion of six residues at, or close to, the first hypervariable region. This has the effect of forcing apart the V_L and V_H regions and increasing the depth and width of the cleft. In the case of λ light-chain dimer studied, one light chain takes on a rotational position corresponding to the 'heavy' chain; the other adopts the light-chain position (Schiffer *et al.*, 1973; Edmundson *et al.*, 1974). The cleft in these dimers is much deeper, forming a funnel with a cavity at the

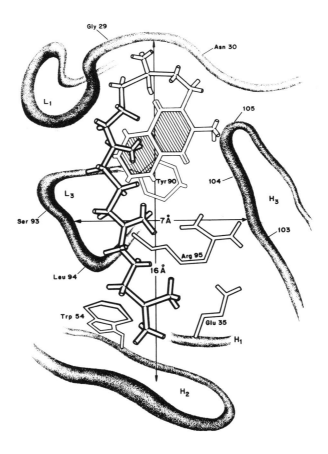

Figure 5 γ-Hydroxy Vitamin K_1 bound to the combining region of the human myeloma IgG molecule NEW. L_1 and L_3 are the first and third light-chain hypervariable regions. (L_2 is deleted in this molecule.) H_1, H_2, and H_3 are the three hypervariable regions of the heavy chain

bottom whose floor is approximately 1·6–1·7 nm below the entrance to the cleft. The κ-chain dimers, Au and Rei, also have a large cavity between the light and 'heavy' chain regions. An important difference in this region is the presence, in Au, of trytophan at position 96 instead of the tyrosine residue found in Rei. The indole ring of this residue protrudes into the cavity, suggesting that it might impede access to a considerable part of the cavity by a moderately large presumptive hapten (Epp et al., 1975; Fehlhammer et al., 1975).

The mouse IgA myeloma, protein 603, binds the small molecule phosphorylcholine approximately in the middle of the cleft. The phosphate moiety touches only the heavy chain at tyrosine 33 and arginine 52. The choline moiety lies at the bottom of the cleft, making contact with residues 102–103 of the heavy chain and residues 91–94 of the light chain; the contact region seems to be composed predominantly of heavy chain and it is of interest that phosphorylcholine-binding myeloma proteins, which do not share the TEPC 15 idiotype, may have light chains that have little resemblance to those found on protein 603 (Poljak, 1975). This suggests that conditions for binding of this small determinant may be relatively non-stringent and are not dependent on a particular light chain, whereas some larger antigens making substantial contact with both light and heavy chains may show a considerable degree of stringency. It is noteworthy that the hypervariable loops form a very extensive region which frames the site of hapten attachment. The third hypervariable region of the heavy chain and the second hypervariable region of the light chain do not make contact with the hapten.

The human IgG myeloma protein NEW binds a γ-hydroxyl derivative of vitamin K_1 (Figure 5) with K_A of $1·7 \times 10^5 \, M^{-1}$. Fab fragment-ligand complexes have been crystallized and analysed by Fourier difference maps (Amzel et al., 1974; Poljak et al., 1974). The vitamin derivative K_1 is a large molecule consisting of a naphthoquinone moiety and a long hydrophobic phytyl side chain. The whole molecule nestles in the cleft, almost completely filling it. The naphthoquinone residue lies obliquely on the floor of the cleft making contact with tyrosine residue 90 of the light chain, with the backbone and side chain of heavy chain residue 104, and with L chain residues 29 and 30. When 2-methyl-1:4-naphthoquinone—the vitamin K molecule without the phytyl tail is bound to protein NEW, it occupies an identical site to that of vitamin derivative K_1 derivative. Of the total binding energy (approximately 7·2 kcal/mole at 20°), the naphthoquinone rings provide approximately 4·2 kcal/mole, thus by difference the phytyl tail provides 3·0 kcal/mole. The phytyl tail loops upward and around, making close contact with the light chain at glycine 29 and asparagine 30. It then proceeds downward and superficially makes contact with the light chain at residues 93 and 94, and with the heavy chain at residue 104. At the free end of the chain, contact is made with a constant heavy-chain tryptophan residue at position 54. Approximately 10–12 amino acid residues make contact with the antigen, and contact is made extensively with both heavy and light chains over a maximal dimension of perhaps 1·5 nm (Amzel et al., 1974; Poljak et al., 1974).

The Mcg λ light-chain dimer appears to have at least three distinct binding sites. One is located on the rim of the funnel-shaped cleft, a second is at the constriction between funnel and cavity, and a third at the bottom of the cavity. These sites bind a whole range of compounds including ε-dansyllysine, colchicine, 1,10-phenanthroline, methadone, morphine, meperidine, 5-acetyluracil, caffeine, theophylline, menadione, and triacetin (Schiffer *et al.*, 1973).

1.9 Conclusions from X-Ray Crystallography and Remaining Problems

Certain general principles are beginning to emerge from the studies so far carried out. These answer, in part, the questions set (see p. 71). It is, however, distinctly possible that further structural elucidation could modify these conclusions.

(*i*) Antigen binding so far observed occurs in the solvent channel between the light- and heavy-chain areas of the V domain. Since only two antigens in actual combining regions have been mapped so far, it is not yet known whether antigen binding is confined to the channel or can extend outside it. Certainly the light-chain dimer model of the combining region suggests that very deep hapten-binding clefts and cavities may exist in some antibodies. More mapping with antibody–antigen complexes will be required before all the region involved in ligation of antigen can be defined.

(*ii*) Analysis of the protein Fab NEW–Vitamin K_1OH complex suggests strongly that antigen binding is not confined to a small, localized contact point, but consists of multipoint contact over an extensive area of the immunoglobulin molecule. This is an observation consistent with the existence of multiple binding sites. If the Mcg model of the immunoglobulin combining region resembles light–heavy chain combining regions, the clustering of binding sites also may be found in antibodies.

(*iii*) It is now clear that both the light and heavy regions as well as the C regions have a common polypeptide fold. Each light and each heavy folded unit has a relatively flat surface which makes contact with the other unit. On assembly each unit makes an angle with the other, that is the two units are not completely symmetrical, but show one dyad axis. At the free end of the Fv domain, the heavy and light chains are not in contact, thus creating a solvent-filled channel. Antigens have been shown to bind to the walls of this channel. The walls of the cleft are composed of six loops, or five in the case of the protein NEW, the tips of which bear hypervariable residues. The nature of the insertions or deletions of amino acid sequence apparently alters the depth of the cleft. For instance, the insertion of six amino acid residues in the first hypervariable loop in κ light chain of the McPc 603 protein forces apart the heavy- and light-chain regions and gives rise to a deeper cleft. From the three-dimensional models, it has been predicted that variations in the length of the third hypervariable loop (around residue 105) would have the same effect. The pattern of amino acid residue variability found at the tips of the loops resembles the pattern of variable or 'permissive' residues found when cytochromes from different species are compared. Here also the loci of greatest variation are found at the tips of outside polypeptide loops. This variability may be permissive in the sense that compensatory change for differences in cleft structure are visible here. It is, however, equally likely that residues at the tips of the loops have some direct functional significance. Haptens appear to bind along the walls of the cleft and not only at the hypervariable residues. The present scanty evidence does not rule out the possibility that the binding region could be much more extensive. It appears that the depth of the cleft can be modulated, exposing new binding sites, and that this may be one method of introducing variability in antigen binding. The light-chain dimers show an extremely wide and deep cleft in which a very large number of determinants binds. Light-chain dimers found in human myelomas show strong affinity for tissue components, infiltrating tissues in the form of amyloid deposits. This effect may be related directly to the large number of combining sites exposed.

(*iv*) It is not clear why antigen binding occurs primarily at the Fab combining region, or why most of the ligand binding observed, for example, in an enzyme molecule such as lysozyme, should occur in the cleft in which the substrate binds. Since it is known that deep cavities are not required for ligand binding in immunoglobulins, a number of crevices, folds, and channels elsewhere in the molecule might be thought to serve equally well. Richards (1974) has considered a similar problem in the case of ribonuclease and has calculated that the atomic packing densities within the substrate-combining cleft are considerably less than at other solvent-exposed regions of the molecule. This suggests that the vibratory modes of various functional groups in the combining region could occur with greater degrees of freedom, and that this may be associated with greater ligating potential. Similar studies carried out with the immunoglobulin molecule would be of great potential interest.

2 RELATIONSHIP BETWEEN ANTIBODY STRUCTURE AND FUNCTION

2.1 Binding Specificity and Amino Acid Sequence

Antibodies of different ligand-binding specificities may have large regions of the primary sequence in common. It is, therefore, reasonable to suggest that in these antibodies those regions which show amino acid sequence variability are those concerned with binding antigens. However, it does not follow from this proposition, that those amino acid residues which show the greatest sequence variability are necessarily the contact residues at which antigens bind. Wu and Kabat (1970) analysed light-chain sequences for variability and plotted variability at each amino acid position *versus* position and obtained a graph showing three regions of greatest sequence variability which they termed 'hypervariable' regions. Capra and Kehoe (1975) performed a similar analysis on heavy-chain variable region sequences and were also able to demonstrate hypervariable regions.

2.2 Groups and Subgroups of the Variable Region

Early studies comparing partial amino acid sequences of different myeloma immunoglobulins showed that if one made an attempt to maximize amino acid residue homology, the variable regions of both the κ and λ light-chain groups could be divided into a number of subgroups. Five human λ (V_λ I–V) and three human κ (V_κ I–III) subgroups have been described (Smith *et al.*, 1971). In the V regions of human heavy chains, three analogous subgroups V_H I–III have been delineated. Similar analyses on mouse κ chains show that the number of subgroups and sub-subgroups is rather large (Hood *et al.*, 1973).

With each group or subgroup, there are amino acid residues which are subgroup specific, (for example, found only in the V_κ I subgroup), group specific (found only in k chains), chain specific (found only in light chains), and species specific (found only in dog light chains).

2.3 Ligand Contact Residues and Hypervariability

Several groups of research workers have compared both monoclonal immunoglobulins and antibody populations of known specificity to see if the amino acid sequence in the hypervariable regions can be correlated with antigen-binding specificity. Cebra *et al.* (1974) have compared the amino acid sequence in the hypervariable regions of guinea-pig anti-DNP and anti-arsonate antibodies, using purified antibodies from strain 13 guinea-pigs. The hypervariable regions were additionally identified by attachment of radioactive affinity reagents. It was found that distinct sequences occur in the hypervariable regions which correlate with DNP binding and other sequences which correlate with the ability to bind arsonate.

Capra *et al.* (1971) examined the light chains from some homogeneous antibodies derived from patients with hypergammaglobulinaemic purpura, all of which had IgG-ligating activity. The amino acid residue sequence are identical in some antibodies up to residue #40; in others there are only infrequent amino acid differences. The hypervariable regions of most of these proteins closely resemble each other.

In contrast to this work is that in which rabbits were hyperimmunized with type VIII staphylococcal polysaccharide. A percentage of such rabbits shows the clonal dominance phenomenon in which the normally heterogeneous antibody becomes highly restricted or monoclonal. Using this phenomenon, a large number of homogeneous rabbit antibodies having specificity for the type VIII staphylococcal polysaccharide has been isolated. These show the normal variations in binding constants for the antigen. The primary structure of a number of V_L and some V_H regions from these monoclonal immunoglobulins has been determined (Margolies *et al.*, 1975). Cluster analysis was carried out using both the specific anti-staphylococcal antibodies and control monoclonal antibodies. A computer was used to search the sequences for groups or clusters of amino acid residues which are consistent within the experimental (anti-type VIII polysaccharide) group and which are different from these sequences in the control group. No such clusters could be demonstrated, suggesting that in the rabbit system many different combining regions contribute to the binding of polysaccharide staphylcoccal.

These results are by no means mutually incompatible. If one considers a set of immunoglobulins on neighbouring branches of an evolutionary tree, these will have diverged from each other only by a few residues. Among the multiple specificities represented in the combining region, it is quite likely that one function will not have been altered by the few amino acid replacements in the V region. Neighbouring branches on such a generic tree will have a set of proteins with V-region structures which closely resemble each other and which have a common antigen-binding specificity.

Since, however, other sets of contact amino acids also may bind the same antigen, several dissimilar sets of immunoglobulins will be distributed widely over non-adjacent branches of the tree since they have no necessary close evolutionary kinship. Depending on the method used for selecting the immuno-globulins, either sets of immunoglobulins with similar or dissimilar V regions can be obtained. It is also conceivable that some antigens may be so stringent in their binding requirements that only one set of evolutionarily related clones on adjacent branches may be able to bind the antigen. In brief, it is a fallacy to believe that, because antibodies with similar V regions bind a common antigen, this antigen can be bound *only* by that type of V region.

2.4 Conservation of Variable Regions

When initial comparisons were made between partial light-chain amino acid sequences in mouse and man, it was noted that more sequence homology exists between certain mouse and human light-chains than between certain V_L-region sequences of two light chains within the species (Smith, 1973). Later work showed great similarity in structure between V regions of inbred and outbred animals of the same species and between the V regions of similar specificity raised in guinea-pigs and mice (Capra and Kehoe, 1974). This similarity is not surprising and may represent, for instance, the retention of certain sequences which ligate some persisting pathogens and thus may be subject to selective pressure. Alternatively, it may represent an example of parallel evolution, or the development of the same lighting sequence from two originally different sequences under the selective pressure exerted by, perhaps, a common pathogen.

2.5 Correlation between Structure and Function

The relationship between primary amino acid sequence in the V region and antibody specificity is, on the one hand, very simple; related structures share specificities. On the other hand, it is very complex, since many different unrelated V regions may bind a single antigenic determinant with different degrees of affinity. It is probably naive to expect to find a common structural feature in the V regions of all antibodies to a small determinant X. There may be several anti-X families which need bear little resemblance to each other, although within each family the members will have close similarities, sharing idiotypes, and perhaps the ability to bind other antigens. The ability to bind X by itself is a poor indication of 'consanguinity' since it is the property of many families of antibodies. A large, site-filling antigen, which requires interaction at several points and demands stringent binding conditions, is more likely to select a smaller set of antibody-producing cell clones, perhaps only one family or even only one clone, which is able to meet these conditions. Similarly non-stringent selection conditions which select for binding of a small determinant over a wide range of binding energies will demand a relatively large heterogeneous collection of antibody-producing cell clones which can meet these non-stringent conditions.

2.6 Polyfunctional Antibody-Combining Regions

In recent years, two lines of evidence have suggested that a single immunoglobulin may have antibody-combining regions which are complementary to several structurally dissimilar antigens. Haimovich and Du Pasquier (1973) have shown that the tadpole has approximately 1×10^6 lymphocytes, yet it is able to mount a specific humoral response against the DNP determinant (anti-DNP). The response to single haptens is usually heterogeneous, involving many different clones of cells which produce anti-DNP antibody. In order that the antibody reaches detectable levels, the number of cells involved in this specific anti-DNP response must be a very considerable proportion of the total. There is no doubt that the tadpole can respond to many antigens, thus there seems to be too few cells at any one time to account for the range of immune responses observed. In addition, clonal-dilution studies, which indicate the presence of many antibodies complementary to one antigenic determinant, have been carried out (Williamson, 1972).

All this work may be summarized by stating that if there is only one anti-hapten specificity per antibody molecule (or per cell), there do not appear to be enough lymphoid cells to account for the number of antigenic specificities. Reciprocally, there appears to be a very large number of clones involved in the production of antibodies against a single haptenic determinant. Over the last decade, homogeneous myeloma proteins which bind antigens have become available and an early finding was that a number of these myeloma proteins can bind more than one haptenic determinant. This binding is competitive, and since only one determinant can be bound at a time to a single combining region, it has been assumed that there are common structural features in the competing determinants that are bound to a single locus on the protein.

Rosenstein and his coworkers (Rosenstein et al., 1972; Jackson and Richards, 1974) examined the combining region of protein 460, a mouse γ A myeloma protein which binds competitively the haptens DNP and menadione. These workers found a sulphydryl group in relation to the combining region. When this group is substituted with a bulky reagent, the ability of protein 460 to bind

DNP   menadione

menadione is impaired, while the ability to bind DNP remains intact. When the protein is partially denatured using 4·3 M guanidine hydrochloride and then allowed to refold partially, the ability to bind DNP is ablated, while menadione binding remains intact. Other methods for differentially affecting one binding activity have been described by these authors.

This work suggests, but does not prove, that there are spatially separated sites within the combining region. Later work on the same protein using the technique of fluorescent energy transfer between donor fluorescent probes placed on the sulphydryl groups and the DNP and menadione molecules bound to their sites shows that there is a minimul separation of 1·2–1·4 nm between the DNP and the menadione binding site (Manjula *et al.*, 1976). To support these findings, dextran bead–spacer–DNP and dextran bead–spacer–menadione columns were constructed with spacer molecules of varying length. The shortest spacer–determinant combination needed to hold protein 460 to the column was determined both for DNP and menadione. The difference in length between the two shortest molecules is 1·25 nm, a finding consistent with the separation distance calculated from the energy transfer experiments (Rosenstein and Richards, 1976). There appears to be reasonable evidence that there is substantial spatial separation between two combining sites within the antibody combining region, making it probable that the combining region is in fact a mosaic of determinant-binding sites.

Even though an individual antibody combining region may bind diverse determinant at different sites, this is not, by itself, proof that multiple binding is physiologically significant. It is, for instance, possible that binding at only one subsite of the V-region cell-surface receptor induces cell proliferation and antibody production. Experiments, however, have shown that this objection does not appear to be true. In rabbits (Varga *et al.*, 1973) and in mice (Varga *et al.*, 1974), isoelectric focusing can pick out individual immunoglobulin bands which bind two dissimilar haptens. In the same animals, the similar double-binding bands can be induced by either of the two antigens (Figure 6), indicating that the binding of both antigens induces cell proliferation and antibody production within the cell clone which binds both antigens (Varga *et al.*, 1973).

Double-binding myeloma proteins appear to have V regions which resemble those of some of the induced antibodies binding the same antigens. Anti-idiotypic sera raised against determinants in the V region of myeloma proteins cross-react with their naturally induced counterparts. They will even do this occasionally

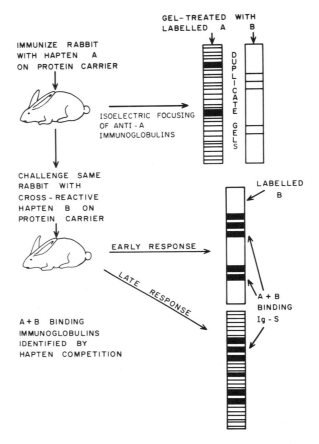

Figure 6 Experimental protocol for determining the presence of immunoglobulins with polyfunctional combining regions in anti-hapten antisera

when the double-binding myeloma proteins arise in one species and the 'natural' double-binding antibodies are induced in another species (Varga *et al.*, 1974), stressing that considerable conservation of the V region between species, or perhaps that parallel evolution, has occurred in the combining region.

It is not yet clear how many different antigens are complementary to a single combining region. It has been estimated that when random antigens are screened, interactions with a K_0 of approximately 1×10^5 M^{-1} occur once in about 140 compounds screened, while weaker interactions in the 1×10^3 M^{-1} range occur much more frequently (once in 20 compounds screened) (Varga, Lande and Richards, 1974). Clearly these figures are only approximate since the choice of antigens can never be really random. Nevertheless, the general principle is that the higher the interaction energy, the less frequently cross-reactions are found. It is intuitively clear that if high energy cross-reactions were very common, antibody populations would be like glue, sticking together all biological structures are showing no population specificity.

The high degree of specificity of an immune serum has been discussed earlier. It has assumed frequently that if a population of antibodies has apparently exclusive specificity for one antigen, the individual antibodies constituting that population must show the same exclusive specificity. In a perceptive article, Talmage (1959) showed that this need not be true and that an apparently highly specific population could be derived from members having different specificities. It is known now that in myeloma proteins individual hapten-combining sites have, in fact, a high degree of specificity and will, for instance, distinguish DNP from mononitrophenols and trinitrophenols (Haimovich and Du Pasquier, 1973). At the same time, protein 460 will bind a number of unrelated haptens at other sites within the combining region. The consequence of this, however, are exactly as Talmage first suggested.

Assuming that a single V region may bind 100 different determinants, if the animal is immunized with determinant A, all those cells producing A-binding immunoglobulins of sufficient affinity will respond to the antigenic stimulus by cell proliferation and antibody production. Thus, all antibody species produced

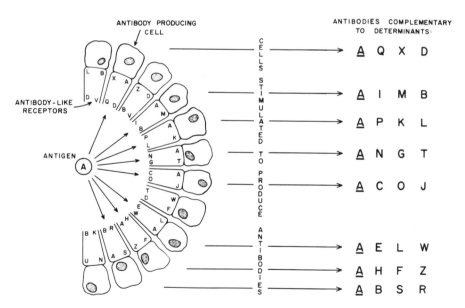

Figure 7 Immune serum specificity as a population phenomenon. Individual B cell receptors are shown as having properties similar to immunoglobulin-combining regions. It is assumed that each is complementary to four different antigens; it is supposed that this figure is in fact much larger. Stimulation by antigen A causes the cells with A specificity to divide and produce antibodies directed against A. The immune serum produced will therefore react in high titre with antigen A. Each immunoglobulin also has other specificities, but because these need not be the same in every molecule, the other specificities, B–Z, will be diluted out and will react only in low titre

bind A. Each antibody will also bind 99 other determinants, but these need not be the same for each antibody and such ligating activity will be present only at a lower level (for example, 1 per cent) in the antibody population and will be diluted out. Thus, antibody specificity is, in essence, a population phenomenon, an average characteristic, rather than the property of each member of the population (see Figure 7).

3 CONCLUSION

In the great complexity of the humoral immune system, a pattern is discernible. Antibody combining regions, although tremendously diverse, are made out of two chains, light and heavy, whose diversity is less than that of the assembled product. Both light and heavy chains give evidence of having evolved over millennia and many of the evolved forms are retained by vertebrates. This retention of many diverse patterns in certain animals serves to create heterogeneous populations of antibodies which as a whole are effective in ligating complex and simple antigens. Combining regions appear to have many common characteristics, judging by the limited number of examples which has so far been analysed. Differences in antibody specificity may depend on quite limited variations in amino acid primary sequence, such as short deletions and insertions which make different parts of the combining region accessible to antigens. The evolutionary process, by numerous step-wise changes of a basic pattern, has created an efficient and adaptable system for combating infection.

ACKNOWLEDGEMENTS

The authors would like to thank the U.S. Public Health Service, the National Science Foundation, and the American Heart Association for their support of this work. This chapter was completed while F.F.R. was a Senior Faculty Fellow of the Josiah Macy Foundation at Glasgow University, Scotland. Most of all, thanks are due to Mrs. Valerie Vishno whose skill and patience in putting together this manuscript is acknowledged with much gratitude.

REFERENCES

Albertson, P., and Phillipson, L. (1960). *Nature (Lond.)*, **185**, 38.
Almeida, J. D., and Waterson, A. P. (1969). *Adv. Virus Res.*, **15**, 307.
Amzel, L. M., Poljak, R. J., Saul, F., Varga, J. M., and Richards, F. F. (1974). *Proc. Nat. Acad. Sci., U.S.A.*, **71**, 1427.

Binz, H., Lindemann, J., and Wigzell, H. (1973). *Nature (Lond.)*, **246**, 146.
Binz, H., Lindemann, J., and Wigzell, H. (1974). In *The Immune System, Genes, Receptors, Signals*, (Sercarz, E. E., Williamson, A. R., and Fox, C. F., eds.), Academic Press, New York and London, 533.
Brient, B. W., Haimovich, J., and Nisonoff, A. (1971). *Proc. Nat. Acad. Sci., U.S.A.*, **68**, 3136.

Capra, J. D., and Kehoe, J. M. (1974). *Proc. Nat. Acad. Sci., U.S.A.*, **71**, 4032.
Capra, J. D., and Kehoe, J. M. (1975). *Adv. Immunol.*, **20**, 1.
Capra, J. D., Winchester, R. J., and Kunkel, H. G. (1971). *Medicine*, **50**, 125.
Cathou, R. E., and Haber, E. (1967). *Biochemistry*, **6**, 513.
Cathou, R. E., Holowka, D. A., and Chan, L. M. (1974). In *Progress in Immunology II*, Vol. I, (Brent, L., and Holborow, J., eds.), North Holland Publishing Co., Amsterdam, p. 63.
Cathou, R. E., and Werner, T. C. (1970). *Biochemistry*, **9**, 3149.
Cebra, J. J., Koo, P. H., and Ray, A. (1974). *Science*, **186**, 263.
Claflin, J. L., and Davie, J. M. (1975). *J. Immunol.*, **114**, 70.
Cohen, S., and Porter, R. R. (1964). *Adv. Immunol.*, **4**, 287.
Converse, C. A., and Richards, F. F. (1968). *Fed. Proc.*, **27**, 683.
Converse, C. A., and Richards, F. F. (1969). *Biochemistry*, **8**, 4431.
Cosenza, H., and Kohler, H. (1972). *Proc. Nat. Acad. Sci., U.S.A.*, **69**, 2701.

Day, E. D. (1972). *Advanced Immuhochemistry*, Williams and Wilkins, Baltimore.
Day, L. A., Sturtevant, J. M., and Singer, S. J. (1963). *Ann. N.Y. Acad. Sci.*, **103**, 611.
Dower, S. K., Dwek, R. A., McLaughlin, A. C., Mole, L. M., Press, E. M., and Sunderland, C. A. (1975). *Biochem. J.*, **149**, 73.
Dwek, R. A., Jones, R., Marsh, D., McLaughlin, A. C., Press, E. M., Price, N. C., and White, A. I. (1975a). *Roy. Soc. Lond., Ser. B*, **272**, 53.
Dwek, R. A., Knott, J. C. A., Marsh, D., McLaughlin, A. C., Press, E. M., Price, N. C., and White, A. I. (1975b). *Eur. J. Biochem.*, **53**, 25.

Edelman, G. M., Cunningham, B. A., Gottlieb, P. D., Rutishauser, U., and Waxdal, M. J. (1969). *Proc. Nat. Acad. Sci., U.S.A.*, **63**, 78.
Edmundson, A. B., Ely, K. R., Girling, R. L., Abola, E. E., Schiffer, M., Westholm, F. A., Fausch, M. D., and Deutsch, H. F. (1974). *Biochemistry*, **13**, 3816.
Eisen, H. N. (1964a). In *Immunology*, Harper and Row, Hagerstown.
Eisen, H. N. (1964b). In *Methods in Medical Research*, (Eisen, H. N., ed.), Vol. 10, Year Book Medical Publishers, Chicago, p. 115.
Eisen, H. N. (1971). In *Progress in Immunology*, Vol. 1, (Amos, B., ed.), Academic Press, New York and London, p. 243.
Eisen, H. N., and Siskind, G. W. (1964). *Biochemistry*, **3**, 996.
Epp, O., Lattman, E. E., Schiffer, M., Huber, R., and Palm, W. (1975). *Biochemistry*, **14**, 4943.

Fehlhammer, H., Schiffer, M., Epp, O., Colman, P. M., Lattman, E. E., Schwager, P., Steigemann, W., and Schramm, H. J. (1975). *Biophys. Struct. Mechan.*, **1**, 139.
Feinstein, A., and Rowe, A. J. (1965). *Nature (Lond.)*, **205**, 147.
Fisher, C. E., and Press, E. M. (1974). *Biochem. J.*, **139**, 135.
Fleet, G. W., Knowles, J. R., and Porter, R. R. (1969). *Nature (Lond.)*, **224**, 511.
Franek, F. (1973). *Eur. J. Biochem.*, **33**, 59.
Freedman, M., Merret, T. R., and Pruzanski, W. (1976). *Immunochemistry*, **13**, 193.

Givol. D. (1974). In *Essays in Biochemistry*, Vol. **10**, Biochemical Society, London, p. 73.
Goetzl, E. J., and Metzger, H. (1970). *Biochemistry*, **9**, 3826.
Green, N. M. (1969). *Adv. Immunol.*, **11**, 1.

Haber, E., Margolies, M. N., Cannon, L. E., and Rosenblatt, M. S. (1975). In *Molecular Approaches to Immunology*, Academic Press, New York and London, p. 303.
Haber, E., and Richards, F. F. (1967). *Proc. Roy. Soc. Lond.*, **166**, 176.
Haber, E., Richards, F. F., Spragg, J., Austen, K. F., Valloton, M., and Page, L. B. (1967). *Cold Spring Harbor Symp. Quant. Biol.*, **32**, 299.

Haber, E., and Stone, M. (1969). *Israel J. Med. Sci.*, **5**, 332.
Haimovich, J., and Du Pasquier, L. (1973). *Proc. Nat. Acad. Sci., U.S.A.*, **70**, 1898.
Haimovich, J., Eisen, H. N., Hurwitz, E., and Givol, D. (1972). *Biochemistry*, **11**, 2389.
Haimovich, J., Givol, D., and Eisen, H. N. (1970). *Proc. Nat. Acad. Sci., U.S.A.*, **67**, 1656.
Haselkorn, D., Friedman, S., Givol, D., and Pecht, I. (1974). *Biochemistry*, **13**, 2210.
Hew, C.-L., Lifter, J., Yoshioka, M., Richards, F. F., and Konigsberg, W. H. (1973). *Biochemistry*, **12**, 4685.
Hochman, J., Inbar, D., and Givol, D. (1973). *Biochemistry*, **12**, 1131.
Hoessli, D., Olander, J., and Little, J. R. (1976). *J. Immunol.*, **113**, 1024.
Hood, L., McKean, D., Farnsworth, V., and Potter, M. (1973). *Biochemistry*, **12**, 741.
Hsia, J. C., and Piette, L. H. (1969). *Archs Biochem. Biophys.*, **129**, 296.

Inbar, D., Hochman, J., and Givol, D. (1972). *Proc. Nat. Acad. Sci., U.S.A.*, **69**, 2659.

Jackson, P., and Richards, F. F. (1974). *J. Immunol.*, **112**, 96.
Jerne, N. K. (1974). *Ann. Immunol. Inst. Pasteur*, **125c**, 373.
Johnston, M. F. M., Barisas, B. G., and Sturtevant, J. M. (1974). *Biochemistry*, **13**, 390.

Kabat, E. A. (1960). *J. Immunol.*, **84**, 82.
Knowles, J. R. (1972). *Ac. Chem. Res.*, **5**, 155.
Kuettner, M. C., Wang, A. L., and Nisonoff, A. (1972). *J. Exp. Med.*, **135**, 579.

Labow, L. W., and Davies, D. R. (1971). *J. Biol. Chem.*, **246**, 3760.
Lafferty, K. J., and Oertelis, S. (1963). *Virology*, **21**, 91.
Lieberman, R., Potter, M., Humphrey, W., Jr., Mushinski, E. B., and Vrana, M. (1975). *J. Exp. Med.*, **142**, 106.
Lieberman, R., Potter, M., Mushinski, E. B., Humphrey, W., Jr., and Rudikoff, S. (1974). *J. Exp. Med.*, **139**, 983.
Lifter, J., Hew, C.-L., Yoshioka, M., Richards, F. F., and Konigsberg, W. H. (1974). *Biochemistry*, **13**, 3567.
Little, J. R., and Eisen, H. N. (1967). *Biochemistry*, **6**, 3119.

Macario, A. J. L., and Conway de Macario, E. (1975). *Curr. Top. Microbiol. Immunol.*, **71**, 125.
Mäkelä, O., and Imanishi, T. (1975). *Eur. J. Immunol.*, **5**, 202.
Manjula, B. N., Richards, F. F., and Rosenstein, R. W. (1976). *Immunochemistry*, **13**, 929.
Margolies, M. N., Cannon, L. E., III, Strosberg, A. D., and Haber, E. (1975). *Proc. Nat. Acad. Sci., U.S.A.*, **372**, 2180.
Metzger, H., and Singer, S. (1963). *Science*, **142**, 674.
Moreno, C., and Kabat, E. A. (1969). *J. Exp. Med.*, **129**, 871.
Murphy, P. D., and Sage, H. J. (1970). *J. Immunol.*, **105**, 460.

Nisonoff, A., Hopper, J. E., and Spring, S. B. (1975). *The Antibody Molecule*, Academic Press, New York and London, p. 448.
Nisonoff, A., and Thorbecke, G. J. (1964). *Ann. Rev. Biochem.*, **33**, 355.
Nisonoff, A., Zappacosta, S., and Jureziz, R. (1967). *Cold Spring Harbor Symp. Quant. Biol.*, **32**, 89.
Noellsen, M. E., Nelson, C. A., Buckley, C. E., III, and Tanford, C. (1965). *J. Biol. Chem.*, **240**, 218.
Northrop, J. A. (1942). *J. Gen. Physiol.*, **25**, 465.

Ohta, Y., Gill, T. J., III, and Leung, C. S. (1970). *Biochemistry*, **9**, 2708.

Padlan, E. A., Segal, D. M., Cohen, G. A., and Davis, D. R. (1974). In *The Immune System, Genes, Receptors, Signals,* (Sercarz, E. E., Williamson, A. R., and Fox, C. F., eds.), Academic Press, New York and London, p. 7.
Painter, R. G., Sage, H. J., and Tanford, C. (1972). *Biochemistry*, **11**, 1327.
Piette, L. H., Kiefer, E. F., Grossberg, A. L., and Pressman, D. (1972). *Immunochemistry*, **9**, 17.
Poljak, R. J. (1975). *Nature (Lond.)*, **256**, 373.
Poljak, R. J., Amzel, L. M., Avey, H. P., Chen, B. L., Phizackerly, R. P., and Saul, F. (1973). *Proc. Nat. Acad. Sci., U.S.A.*, **70**, 3305.
Poljak, R. J., Amzel, L. M., Chen, B. L., Phizackerley, R. P., and Saul, F. (1974). *Proc. Nat. Acad. Sci., U.S.A.*, **71**, 3440.
Porter, R. R. 1958). *Nature (Lond.)*, **182**, 670.
Porter, R. R., and Press, E. M. (1962). *Ann. Rev. Biochem.*, **31**, 621.
Potter, M., and Lieberman, R. (1970). *J. Exp. Med.*, **132**, 737.

Reichlin, M. (1974). *Immunochemistry*, **11**, 21.
Richards, F. F. (1974). *J. Mol. Biol.*, **82**, 1.
Richards, F. F., Konigsberg, W. H., Rosenstein, R. W., and Varga, J. M. (1975). *Science, N.Y.*, **187**, 130.
Richards, F. F., Lifter, J., Hew, C.-L., Yoshioka, M., and Konigsberg, W. H. (1974). *Biochemistry*, **13**, 3572.
Richards, F. F., Sloane, R. W., Jr., and Haber, E. (1967). *Biochemistry*, **6**, 476.
Rosenstein, R. W., Musson, R. A., Armstrong, M. Y. K., Konigsberg, W. H., and Richards, F. F. (1972). *Proc. Nat. Acad. Sci., U.S.A.*, **69**, 877.
Rosenstein, R. W., and Richards, F. F. (1976). *Immunochemistry*, **13**, 939.
Rubinstein, W. A., and Little, J. R. (1970). *Biochemistry*, **9**, 2106.
Ruoho, A. E., Kiefer, H., Roeder, P. E., and Singer, S. J. (1973). *Proc. Nat. Acad. Sci., U.S.A.*, **70**, 2567.

Schechter, B., Schechter, I., and Sela, M. (1970). *J. Biol. Chem.*, **245**, 1438.
Schiffer, M., Girling, R. L., Ely, K. R., and Edmundson, A. B. (1973). *Biochemistry*, **12**, 4620.
Schlessinger, J., Steinberg, I. Z., Givol, D., Hochman, J., and Pecht, I. (1975). *Proc. Nat. Acad. Sci., U.S.A.*, **72**, 2775.
Segal, D., Padlan, E. A., Cohen, G. H., Rudikoff, S., Potter, M., and Davies, D. R. (1974). *Proc. Nat. Acad. Sci., U.S.A.*, **71**, 4298.
Singer, S. J., and Doolittle, R. F. (1966). *Science, N.Y.*, **153**, 13.
Sirisinha, S., and Eisen, H. N. (1971). *Proc. Nat. Acad. Sci., U.S.A.*, **68**, 3130.
Smith, G. P. (1973). *The Variation and Adaptive Expression of Antibodies.* Harvard University Press, Cambridge, Mass.
Smith, G. P., Hood, L., and Fitch, W. M. (1971). *Ann. Rev. Biochem.*, **40**, 969.
Smith, R. A. G., and Knowles, J. R. (1973). *J. Am. Chem. Soc.*, **95**, 5072.
Steiner, L. A., and Eisen, H. N. (1966). *Bacteriol. Rev.*, **30**, 383.
Steiner, L. A., and Eisen, H. N. (1967a). *J. Exp. Med.*, **126**, 1161.
Steiner, L. A., and Eisen, H. N. (1967). *J. Exp. Med.*, **126**, 1185.
Stevenson, G. T. (1973). *Biochem. J.*, **133**, 827.
Steward, M. W., and Petty, R. E. (1972). *Immunology*, **23**, 881.
Stryer, L., and Griffith, O. H. (1965). *Proc. Nat. Acad. Sci., U.S.A.*, **54**, 1785.

Talmage, D. W. (1959). *Science*, **129**, *Immunochemistry*, **12**, 173.

Utsumi, S., and Karush, F. (1964). *Biochemistry*, **3**, 1329.

Valentine, R. C., and Green, N. M. (1967). *J. Mol. Biol.*, **27**, 615.

Varga, J. M., Konigsberg, W. H., and Richards, F. F. (1973). *Proc. Nat. Acad. Sci., U.S.A.*, **70**, 3269.

Varga, J. M., Lande, S., and Richards, F. F. (1974). *J. Immunol.*, **112**, 1565.

Varga, J. M., Rosenstein, R. W., and Richards, F. F. (1974). *Fed. Proc.*, **33**, 810.

Vaughan, R. J., and Westheimer, F. H. (1969). *J. Am. Chem. Soc.*, **91**, 217.

Waxdal, M. J., Konigsberg, W. H., and Edelman, G. M. (1968). *Biochemistry*, **7**, 1967.

Weil, E., and Felix, A. (1916). *Wien. Klin. Wochenschr.*, **29**, 974.

Weltman, J. K., and Edelman, G. M. (1967). *Biochemistry*, **6**, 1437.

Williamson, A. R. (1972). *Biochem. J.*, **130**, 325.

Wiswesser, W. J. (1973). *Aldrichim. Acta*, **6**, 41.

Wofsy, L., Metzger, H., and Singer, S. J. (1962). *Biochemistry*, **1**, 1031.

Wofsy, L., and Parker, D. A. (1967). *Cold Spring Harbor Symp. Quant. Biol.*, **32**, 111.

Wu, T. T., and Kabat, E. A. (1970). *J. Exp. Med.*, **132**, 211.

Ygerabide, J., Epstein, H. F., and Stryer, L. (1970). *J. Mol. Biol.*, **51**, 573.

Yoo, T. J., Roholt, O. A., and Pressman, D. (1967). *Science, N.Y.*, **157**, 707.

Yoshioka, M., Lifter, J., Hew, C.-L., Converse, C. A., Armstrong, M. Y. K., Konigsberg, W. H., and Richards, F. F. (1973). *Biochemistry* **12**, 4679.

CHAPTER 7

Affinity of the Antibody—Antigen Reaction and its Biological Significance

M. W. Steward

1 INTRODUCTION

The interaction of antibody and antigen has been studied widely at both the qualitative and quantitative levels. Qualitative analysis of the antibody–antigen reaction in kinetic and thermodynamic terms has provided considerable information as to the nature of this reaction. It is clear from these observations that for an understanding of the antibody–antigen reaction and its functional significance in biology an appreciation of the importance of antibody affinity is essential. Karush (1970) has expressed this view in the following way: 'the measurement of antibody affinity and the recognition of its decisive role in the biological activities of the antibody molecule have brought a new dimension to our understanding and exploration of the immune response'. In this discussion of the antibody–antigen reaction, particular emphasis will be given to a consideration of antibody affinity and its biological significance.

2 FORCES INVOLVED IN THE ANTIBODY–ANTIGEN REACTION

The interaction of antibody and antigen at equilibrium may be expressed in the following way

$$\text{Ab} + \text{Ag} \underset{k_d}{\overset{k_a}{\rightleftharpoons}} \text{Ab–Ag} \tag{1}$$

where Ab represents free antibody; Ag, free antigen; Ab–Ag, the antibody–antigen complex; k_a and k_d, the association and dissociation constants, respectively.
Applying the law of mass action to this interaction,

$$k_a[\text{Ab}][\text{Ag}] = k_d[\text{Ab–Ag}] \tag{2}$$

thus the equilibrium constant or affinity (K) may be calculated

$$\frac{k_a}{k_d} = K = \frac{[\text{Ab–Ag}]}{[\text{Ab}][\text{Ag}]}$$

The intermolecular forces which contribute to the stabilization of the complex are the same as those involved in the stabilization of the specific configuration of proteins and other macromolecules. Antibody affinity may be considered therefore as the summation of attractive and repulsive non-covalent intermolecular forces resulting from the interaction of the antibody binding site and the homologous antigenic determinant.

2.1 Hydrogen Bonding

Hydrogen bonds result from the interaction of an hydrogen atom covalently linked to an electronegative atom with the unshared electron pair of a second electronegative atom. The hydrogen donor and acceptor atoms are usually strongly electronegative, and in antibody–antigen reactions, amino and hydroxyl groups are involved predominantly. The contribution of this type of bond for the stabilization of the antibody–antigen complex is small, particularly in view of the competitive effect of an aqueous polar solvent environment.

2.2 Apolar or Hydrophobic Bonding

The interaction of apolar or hydrophobic molecules with an aqueous environment is of particular importance in antibody–antigen reactions. Apolar or hydrophobic bonding occurs as a result of the preference of such groups for self-association so that their extent of contact with water decreases. In this way, a lower energy state is achieved with a concomitant increase in entropy, resulting in a net attractive force. Hydrophobic bonding is an entropy driven, endothermic process, and the strength of such interactions increases with temperature.

2.3 Ionic or Coulombic Interaction

This attractive force is the result of the interaction of oppositely charged ionic groups such as an ionized amino group (NH_3^+) and an ionized carboxyl group (COO^-). While it is clear that an inverse relationship exists between the charge on an immunogen and the charge on the antibody it induces, these coulombic interactions do not appear to play a prominent role in the stabilization of the antibody–antigen complex.

2.4 Van der Waals Interactions

These forces result from the interaction of the electron clouds of polar groups. This interaction involves the induction of oscillating dipoles in the two molecules concerned and results in an attractive force. The greater the complementarity of the electron clouds of the two groups concerned, the closer will be the association of the two molecules, resulting in an increased attractive force.

2.5 Steric Repulsive Forces

The attractive forces discussed so far all increase as the distance between the interacting groups decreases. The coulombic forces are inversely proportional to the square of this distance and Van der Waals forces are inversely proportional to the sixth power of this distance. Steric repulsion, on the other hand, is more sensitive to distance and varies inversely with the twelfth power of the distance between the interacting groups. The repulsive force between non-bonded atoms arises from the interpenetration of their respective electron clouds and therefore the closer the complementarity of the electron cloud shapes, the lower will be the repulsive force. In the antibody–antigen reaction this force therefore governs the degree to which an antigenic determinant can fit into the binding site of the antibody. A non-homologous antigenic determinant will not have an electron cloud which is complementary to that of the various groups defining the antibody binding site and thus the repulsive force will be high and the attractive forces will be minimized. In this way, the antibody will exhibit a low affinity for the particular antigenic determinant. Conversely, where the electron clouds of the antigenic determinant and antibody combining site are complementary, steric repulsion will be minimized and the attractive forces maximized resulting in a high affinity antibody–antigen interaction. Steric repulsive forces may be viewed, therefore, as providing the basis for antibody specificity in its selective interaction with a specific antigenic determinant.

3 THERMODYNAMIC ASPECTS OF THE ANTIBODY–ANTIGEN REACTION

The law of mass action plays a central role in the derivation of equations for thermodynamic affinity measurement. This subject has been reviewed recently in detail by Day (1972), thus only a brief discussion will be included here.

For thermodynamic measurement of antibody affinity, it is necessary for the reactants, both antibody and antigen, to be pure and in solution. In addition, the reactants should be homogeneous with regard to antigenic determinants and antibody binding sites for ideal affinity measurement. In practice, however, such ideal situations do not exist; antibodies are notoriously heterogeneous, particularly with regard to their structure, and also exhibit multivalence for antigen. However, in spite of these limitations, reasonably precise affinity measurements can be made using purified antibodies to defined monovalent haptens. The experimental determination of antibody-bound hapten and free hapten at equilibrium over a range of free hapten concentrations, followed by the analysis of the data by the equation presented below form the basis of affinity measurements.

From the application of the law of mass action to the antibody–antigen reaction (Equation (2)) a form of the Langmuir Adsorption isotherm may be derived

$$\frac{[Ab–Ag]}{[Ab]} = r = \frac{nK[Ag]}{1 + K[Ag]} \tag{3}$$

where r is the moles of antigen (hapten) bound per mole of antibody; $[Ab–Ag]$, bound antibody concentration; $[Ab]$, free antibody concentration; $[Ag]$, free hapten concentration; n, antibody valence; and K, equilibrium constant or affinity.
From Equation (3)

$$\frac{r}{[Ag]} = nK - rK \tag{4}$$

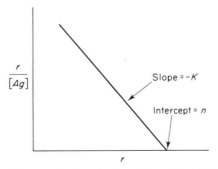

Figure 1 Scatchard plot of ideal antibody–antigen binding

Therefore a plot of $r/[Ag]$ *versus* r over a range of free hapten concentrations (Scatchard, 1949) allows values of antibody affinity (K) and antibody valence to be derived (see Figure 1). For divalent anti-hapten antibody (where $n = 2$) Equation (4) can be used to calculate the average intrinsic association constant K_0 of the antibody for the hapten. When half the antibody binding sites are bound ($r = 1$), then

$$\frac{r}{[Ag]} = nK - rK$$

becomes

$$\frac{1}{[Ag]} = 2K - K = K_0$$

Therefore K_0 is equal to the reciprocal of the free hapten concentration at equilibrium when half the antibody sites are hapten-bound.

Antibody affinity also may be calculated by the Langmuir plot (Figure 2) using the following equation derived from Equations (3) or (4):

$$\frac{1}{r} = \frac{1}{n} \cdot \frac{1}{[Ag]} \cdot \frac{1}{K} + \frac{1}{n} \tag{5}$$

For ideal antibody–antigen binding both Scatchard and Langmuir equations should give rise to linear plots. However, even when using isolated and purified anti-hapten antibody, their plots deviate from linearity. The reason for this deviation has been ascribed to the existence of heterogeneity of antibody affinities within an antibody population. The existence of such heterogeneity has been known for many years, Pauling *et al.* (1944), Karush (1956) and Heidelberger and Kendall (1935), have shown that the distribution of affinities in an antibody population can be described in terms of a Gaussian error function. Similarly, Nisonoff and Pressman (1958) have shown that affinity distribution can be described by the closely related Sipsian distribution function (Sips, 1948)

$$\frac{r}{n} = \frac{[K_0 Ag]^a}{1 + [K_0 Ag]^a}$$

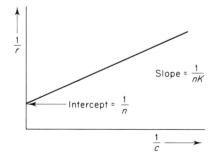

Figure 2 Langmuir plot of ideal antibody–antigen binding

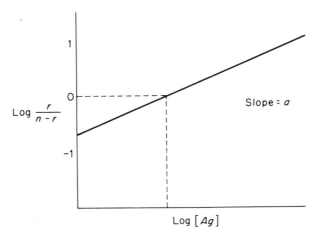

Figure 3 Sips plot of ideal antibody–antigen binding. The graphical determination of average intrinsic association constant (K_0) and heterogeneity index (a)

Karush (1962), utilizing the logarithmic transformation of the Sips' equation

$$\log \frac{r}{n - r} = a \log K_0 + a \log [Ag]$$

has demonstrated that a plot of $\log r/(n - r)$ *versus* $\log$ Ag yields a straight line where the index of heterogeneity (a) is given by the slope (Figure 3). As the heterogeneity index approaches 1·0 the antibody population approaches homogeneity with regard to association constants. Furthermore, K_0, the average intrinsic association constant, is given by $1/[Ag]$ where $\log r/(n - r) = 0$ and is thus the peak of the presumed normal distribution (Figure 3). While this type of analysis of antibody–hapten binding data represents a convenient approximation of the true situation, Pressman *et al.* (1970) have challenged the assumption that there is a continuous heterogenous population of antibodies with affinities following a Gaussian distribution. They have suggested the existence of limited heterogeneity, in which the majority of the antibody population is composed of a limited number of types of antibody with different affinities. Medof and Aladjem (1971) also have reported that the distribution of affinities could not be approximated to a Gaussian or Sipsian distribution. Werblin and Siskind (1972) demonstrated that DNP–anti-DNP binding data plotted according to the Sips' equation are not linear, suggesting that the distribution of affinities is actually asymmetric. These authors confirmed the existence of an asymmetrical distribution of affinities by the use of iterative computational techniques to generate approximate affinity distributions from the experimental binding data. In this way, it was shown that only in rabbit anti-DNP serum obtained seven days after immunization with DNP–BGG in Freund's complete adjuvant was the distribution of affinities approximately symmetrical. In serum obtained at intervals for up to one year after immunization, the distribution of affinities became progressively more asymmetrical.

The non-linearity of Sipsian binding curves and the asymmetrical distribution of affinities therefore challenges the assumption that K_0 (average intrinsic affinity) precisely describes the affinity characteristics of a given antibody population. The non-linearity of binding curves clearly means that the slope will differ at various parts of the curve. Accordingly, values of K_0 and a, calculated with the assumption of linearity, will differ depending on the portion of the binding curve used. The conclusion to be drawn from these studies is that while average affinity values calculated by the assumption of a Gaussian or Sipsian distribution of affinities are relatively easy to obtain, and are satisfactory for many purposes, the handling of binding data by more complex methods, such as described by Werblin and Siskind (1972), is required for a more precise description of the distribution of affinity. More recently, Mukkur *et al.* (1974) have described a simpler, graphical method for determining the *total* affinity constant, K_t which represents the sum of the weighted affinities of the antibody subpopulations in an antibody preparation. K_t values obtained graphically are in close agreement to those determined by computer calculation.

It will be clear from the preceding discussion that measurement of K_0 requires a precise knowledge of the total amount of antibody present in the system. This poses several difficulties, particularly since there is no completely suitable method for determining the amount of antibody. The traditional method of precipitin analysis has the obvious limitation that non-precipitating antibody will not be detected. Furthermore, there is evidence that antibodies of differing affinities have different precipitating characteristics (Morgan *et al.*, unpublished observations). Antibody purification procedures involving adsorption onto and elution from antigen immunoadsorbents provide 'pure' antibody preparations, but the possibility of selection for antibodies of a particular affinity cannot be ruled out. Thus, for many purposes, this type of procedure is not suitable. In situations where isolation and purification of antibody is not possible or is not desirable, the calculation of affinity can be made with respect to total antibody binding sites (Ab_t) rather than to antibody concentration and valence (Nisonoff and Pressman, 1958). Equation (5) is thus rewritten as

$$\frac{1}{b} = \frac{1}{Ab_t} \cdot \frac{1}{[Ag]} \cdot \frac{1}{K} + \frac{1}{Ab_t}$$

where b is bound antigen and Ab_t the total antibody binding sites. Therefore, in this procedure, the antibody binding site concentration is determined by saturation of the total sites by high concentrations of free antigen. Thus, in a plot $1/b$ *versus* $1/[Ag]$, when $1/[Ag] = 0$, then $1/b = 1/Ab_t$. The value for Ab_t is obtained graphically by extrapolation of the binding curve to infinite free antigen concentration. This method also is not without its serious limitations. Firstly, saturation of low-affinity antibody binding sites requires high concentrations of antigen. In addition, graphical extrapolation to infinite free antigen concentration is a particularly uncertain procedure when heterogeneous antibody

240

populations are being studied. Relatively small errrors in the estimation of Ab_t can give rise to considerable errors in the subsequent calculation of an affinity value. Therefore, the measurement of antibody binding sites is an operationally defined concept and at best gives an arbitrary definition of the amount of antibody. It still remains as an important limitation to a fuller understanding of the thermodynamics of the antibody–antigen reaction.

Alternative approaches to the measurement of the affinity of antibody populations, which do not involve direct estimation of antibody level, have been proposed. Celada *et al.* (1969) described an empirical relationship between antibody dilution and antigen concentration which provides an estimate of an index of avidity* of the antiserum

$$\log \mu l \text{ antiserum} = m + s \log \mu g \text{ Ag}$$

where μl antiserum is the volume of antiserum required to bind 50 per cent of the antigen added, Ag; s is the slope and represents the index of avidity; and m is the intercept on the ordinate when $\log \mu g$ Ag $= 0$. The slope (s) of the plot of log volume of antiserum required to bind half the added antigen *versus* log amount of antigen added varies between 0 and 1, and has been shown to correlate with affinity values determined by other methods (Schirrmacher, 1972; Steward and Petty, 1972a; Ahlstedt *et al.*, 1973). Taylor (1975), in a detailed mathematical appraisal of this method, has suggested that while for biological reasons, s is generally correlated with affinity K_0, it is not mathematically dependent upon K_0 but depends on the distribution of antibody subpopulations of different affinity within the antiserum.

Recently, Paul and Elfenbein (1975) have reported a technique for the determination of affinity which is independent of a measurement of total antibody, based on the antigen capacity method of Farr (1958). The following expression was derived

$$K = \frac{R(B/F)_x \cdot B_i - (B/F)_i \cdot B_x}{(1 - R)B_i \cdot B_x}$$

in which $R = ABC_x/ABC_i$ where ABC_i and ABC_x refer to the antigen binding capacity (concentration of antigen bound × serum dilution) with the index concentration i of antigen and a lower concentration of antigen x, respectively. B_i and B_x refer to bound antigen at the two antigen concentrations. These authors demonstrated that for myeloma anti-DNP antibody, this method yields unambiguous values for K_t which compare well with those determined by equilibrium dialysis. They pointed out that for heterogeneous antibody populations, the estimated value for K varies according to the value of R—that is K

* In the literature, *affinity* and *avidity* commonly are used synonymously. However, it is now accepted generally that the term *affinity* is a thermodynamic expression of the primary binding energy of an antibody binding site for an antigenic determinant. Experimentally, this term has its most precise application in monovalent hapten–anti-hapten systems. *Avidity*, on the other hand, although it is dependent on affinity, also involves other contributing factors such as antibody valence, antigenic valence, and factors associated with binding, but not concerned directly with the primary antibody–antigen interaction.

increases as the fraction of antibody binding sites bound falls. These observations are consistent with those of Werblin and Siskind (1972) using anti-hapten antibody and of Steward and Petty (1972a) using anti-protein antibody, illustrating that because of antibody heterogeneity, affinity values obtained depend upon the region of the binding curve employed for calculation. Thus, although this procedure overcomes the problem of antibody site determination, the problem of heterogeneity of antibody affinities remains and the value of K obtained is not an average intrinsic association constant.

Antibody heterogeneity and the adequate measurement of the level of the antibody are two problems which have put considerable constraint on the understanding of the thermodynamics of the antibody–antigen reaction. Nevertheless, using the methods described above, workers in several laboratories have been able to make significant contributions to the available knowledge of this aspect of the immune response.

4 KINETIC ASPECTS OF THE ANTIBODY–ANTIGEN REACTION

It has been known for many years that antibody–antigen reactions occur rapidly (Hooker and Boyd, 1935), and it is this speed of reaction which has made kinetic studies difficult when traditional kinetic methods are employed. Utilizing concentrations of reactants necessary for efficient measurement, the time of mixing is the rate-limiting step and equilibration occurs before any changes in concentration can be determined as a function of time. Furthermore, kinetic data obtained with complex antigens proved to be difficult to interpret (Goldberg and Campbell, 1951). However, the application of more sophisticated techniques and instrumentation to the study not of a complex antigen–antibody system but rather of the simple hapten–anti-hapten reaction

$$Ab + H \xrightleftharpoons[k_{2,1}]{k_{1,2}} Ab-H$$

has broadened our knowledge of the kinetics of this reaction. The use of techniques for the study of fast reactions such as the temperature-jump relaxation method (Eigen and DeMaeyer, 1963) and the stopped-flow technique (Chance, 1963), in combination with sensitive spectrophotometric methods for the measurement of hapten binding has provided an opportunity to make meaningful kinetic measurements of the antibody–antigen reaction.

A concise account of the principle and application of both the stopped-flow and the temperature-jump relaxation techniques has been given recently by Froese and Sehon (1971, 1975). In brief, the stopped-flow technique consists of forcing the reactants at high volocity into a reaction chamber and monitoring spectrophotometric changes with time using an oscilloscope. In this way, data for the calculation of the association rate constant $k_{1,2}$ are obtained. In the temperature-jump technique, the antigen–antibody system under study is allowed to reach equilibrium. The equilibrium is then disturbed by a sudden change in temperature of five to 10°C achieved by the discharge of a high-voltage

Table 1 Hapten–antihapten rate constants

Antibody	Hapten	$k_{1,2}$ $(M^{-1} sec^{-1})$	$k_{2,1}$ (sec^{-1})	K_0† (M^{-1})	Reference
Rabbit anti-DNP	DNP-lysine (i)	8.4×10^7	11‡	7.7×10^7	Day et al. (1963)
Mouse anti-DNP*	DNP-lysine (ii)	1.1×10^7	0.5‡	2.2×10^7	Kelly et al. (1971)
"	DNP-lysine (iii)	1.3×10^8	53	2.0×10^6	Pecht et al. (1972a)
Rabbit anti-DNP	DNP-glycine	1.9×10^8	1300	—	Pecht et al. (1972b)
"	DNP-aminocaproate	9.7×10^7	1.1‡	9.1×10^7	Day et al. (1963)
"	DNP-aminocaproate	8.0×10^7	8.7	—	Barisas et al. (1975)
"	TNP-aminocaproate	4.0×10^7	270	—	Barisas et al. (1975)
"	1N-3,6S-2-DNP	8.0×10^7	1.4‡	5.9×10^7	Day et al. (1963)
"	1N-2,5S-4-DNP*	9.5×10^6	76	1.5×10^5	Kelly et al. (1971)
"	1N-2,5S-4-DNP†	1.6×10^7	80	1.5×10^5	Froese (1968)
"	1N-2,5S-4-pNP	1.4×10^7	410	1.0×10^4	Froese (1968)
Rabbit anti-TNP	TNP-aminocaproate	9.0×10^7	1.6	—	Barisas et al. (1975)
"	DNP-aminocaproate	7.5×10^7	6.7	—	Barisas et al. (1975)
Rabbit anti-p-nitrophenyl	DHNDS–NP	1.8×10^8	760	5.8×10^5	Froese and Sehon (1965)
Rabbit anti-p-azobenzenearsonate	N–R'	2.0×10^7	50	—	Froese et al. (1962)
"	DMP–R'	1.1×10^7	1.4×10^{-3}	—	Ferber (1965)
Bovine anti-ADHB†	ADHB	6.2×10^8	6000	—	Haustein (1971)
Rabbit anti-fluorescein	Fluorescein	4.0×10^8	5.0×10^{-3}	6.5×10^{10}	Levison (1971)
Sheep anti-digoxin	Digoxin	1.7×10^7	3.4×10^{-4}	1.9×10^{10}	Smith and Skubitz (1975)
Rabbit anti-ouabain	Ouabain	1.3×10^7	6.4×10^{-3}	3.5×10^9	Smith and Skubitz (1975)
"	"	8.0×10^6	1.5×10^{-3}	3.5×10^9	Skubitz and Smith (1975)

DNP, 2,4-dinitrophenyl; TNP, 2,4,6-trinitrophenyl; 1N-3,6S-2-DNP, 1-hydroxy-2-(2,4-dinitrophenylazo)-3,6 naphthalene disulphonate; 1N-2,5S-4 DNP, 1-hydroxy-4-(2,4-dinitrophenylazo)-2,5-naphthalene disulphonate; 1N-2,5S-4-pNP, 1-hydroxy-4-(p-nitrophenylazo)-2,5-naphthalene disulphonate; DHNDS–NP, 4,5-dihydroxy-3-(p-nitrophenylazo)-2,7-naphthalene disulphonate; N–R', 1-naphthol-4-[4-(4'-azobenzeneazo) phenylarsonate]; DMP–R', p(p-dimethyl-aminophenylazo)-benzenearsonate: ADHB, 4-(3-aminophenyl)-2,6-diphenyl-pyridinium-N-(4-hydroxyphenyl)-betaine

* Mouse myeloma (MOPC 315) IgA protein with anti-DNP activity
† Calculated from $k_{2,1} = k_{1,2}/K_0$
‡ Determined by equilibrium measurement
Data, in part, from Froese and Sehon (1975), with permission

condenser. The re-equilibration of the system is followed as a function of time using an oscilloscope. From the trace, the relaxation time τ may be determined. The relationship between relaxation time and the rate constants of the new equilibrium is given by the expression

$$\frac{1}{\tau} = k_{2,1} + k_{1,2} \left[(Ab) + (H) \right]$$

where (Ab) and (H) are the equilibrium concentrations of antibody sites and hapten, respectively. The slope and intercept of a plot of $1/\tau$ versus $[(Ab) + (H)]$ give the values for $k_{1,2}$ and $k_{2,1}$, respectively. Recently, Skubitz and Smith (1975) have described a simplified technique for the determination of $k_{1,2}$ and $k_{2,1}$, using dextran-coated charcoal to determine antibody-bound and free hapten. The specific activity of the hapten is sufficiently high to allow the use of concentrations of reactants (10^{-10}–10^{-9} M) well below those at which mixing is the rate-limiting step. The data are analysed by first-order and pseudo-second-order treatments.

The work of several authors using the stopped-flow and temperature-jump techniques has shown that the value for $k_{1,2}$ is approximately the same for all antibody–hapten systems tested; all the values obtained are within one order of magnitude of 10^8 M^{-1} sec^{-1}. On the other hand, a great variation in the dissociation rate constants k_{21} has been observed (Table 1). Froese (1968) demonstrated that a 10-fold difference in the average association constant k_0 of anti-DNP antibody for two cross-reacting haptens is due to differences in $k_{2,1}$ rather than to $k_{1,2}$ (Table 2) and suggested that the stability of the antibody–hapten complex was governed by the dissociation rate constant. These results plus those of others (Haselkorn et al., 1971; Pecht et al., 1972a, b; Barisas et al., 1975; Skubitz and Smith, 1975; Smith and Skubitz, 1975) have confirmed that it is $k_{2,1}$ that determines the affinity of antibody for hapten.

Table 2 Kinetic and equilibrium measurements of anti-DNP antibody reacting with two cross-reacting haptens

Hapten	$k_{1,2}$(M^{-1} sec^{-1})	$k_{2,1}$(sec^{-1})	$K = k_{1,2}/k_{2,1}$ (M^{-1})	K_0(M^{-1})‡
1N–2,5S–4–DNP*	$1\cdot6 \times 10^7$	80	$2\cdot0 \times 10^5$	$1\cdot5 \times 10^5$
1N–2,5S–4–pNP†	$1\cdot4 \times 10^7$	410	$3\cdot4 \times 10^4$	1×10^4

* hydroxy-4-(2,4-dinitrophenylazo)-2,5-naphthalene disulphonate
† 1-hydroxy-4-(p-nitrophenylazo)-2-5-naphthalene disulphonate
‡ From equilibrium data
Data from Froese (1968). Reproduced by permission of Pergamon Press and the author

5 EXPERIMENTAL PROCEDURES FOR DETERMINING ANTIBODY AFFINITY

Several techniques are currently available for estimating the affinity and avidity of antibodies. Thermodynamic estimations of affinity essentially involve

Table 3 Methods for the measurement of the affinity and kinetics of the antibody–antigen reaction

Method	Principal applicable antigens	Parameter measured	Reference
Equilibrium dialysis	Haptens, dialysable antigens	Affinity	Eisen (1964)
Fluorescence quenching ⎱ Fluorescence enhancement ⎰	Haptens and antigens with specific fluorescence properties	Affinity	Velick et al. (1960) / Parker et al. (1967)
Fluorescence polarization	Haptens, proteins	Affinity / Avidity	Dandliker et al. (1964)
Ammonium sulphate globulin precipitation	Haptens, antigens soluble in 50 per cent saturated ammonium sulphate	Affinity / Avidity	Stupp et al. (1969) / Steward and Petty (1972b) / Gaze et al. (1973)
Dextra-coated charcoal	Protein antigens	Avidity index	Celada et al. (1969)
Antiglobulin precipitation	Haptens / Haptens, proteins, carbohydrates	Affinity / Affinity, Avidity	Herbert et al. (1965) / Steward and Petty (1972b)
Equilibrium molecular sieving	Haptens, proteins, carbohydrates	Affinity / Avidity	Stone and Metzger (1968)
Ultracentrifugation	Proteins	Avidity	Normansell (1970)
Phage neutralization	Haptens	Avidity	Mäkelä (1966)
Equilibrium filtration	Viruses	Avidity	Fazekas de St. Groth (1961)
Haemolysin transfer	Erythrocytes	Relative avidity	Taliaferro et al. (1959)
Plaque-forming cell avidity	Haptens, proteins	Avidity	Andersson (1970)
Association and dissociation rate measurement			
Ammonium sulphate	Antigens soluble in 50 per cent saturated ammonium sulphate	$k_{1,2}$ $k_{2,1}$	Talmage (1960)
Dextran-coated charcoal	Haptens with high specific radioactivity	$k_{1,2}$ $k_{2,1}$	Skubitz and Smith (1975)
Stopped-flow technique	Haptens	$k_{1,2}$	Chance (1963)
Temperature-jump relaxation technique	Haptens	$k_{1,2}$ $k_{2,1}$	Eigen and De Meyer (1963)

the determination of the concentration of free and bound antigen under equilibrium conditions using techniques that do not disturb the equilibrium. In general, the separation of antibody-bound and free antigen is achieved either by dialysis, selective precipitation, or gel filtration, or by utilizing changes in the properties of the antigen or antibody, such as fluorescence, occurring as a result of binding. The kinetic approaches to the measurement of affinity have been described above. Other techniques applicable to avidity measurement at the antibody-forming cell level and to highly complex antigens such as erythrocytes also have been described. The various techniques are listed in Table 3, together with pertinent references.

6 THE BIOLOGICAL SIGNIFICANCE OF ANTIBODY AFFINITY

6.1 The Role of Antibody Polyvalence

The average intrinsic association constant, K_0, for the interaction of an antibody binding site with a monovalent antigen (intrinsic affinity) is clearly of both conceptual and experimental importance. However, in view of the polyvalence of antibody molecules, it is obvious that in biological terms it is unlikely that intrinsic affinity adequately describes the interaction of antibody and polyvalent antigen.

The term 'functional affinity' has been used to describe the energy of interaction of the antibody combining sites with the antigenic determinants on a polyvalent antigen—(avidity, see p. 240). Since naturally occurring antigens such as viruses and bacteria have repeating antigenic structures on their surfaces, it is clear that in immune responses to infection *in vivo* it is the functional rather than intrinsic infinity of the antibody which is important. Several years ago, Burnet *et al.* (1937) speculated that bivalent attachment of antibody to a viral particle would be energetically more advantageous than monovalent binding. Recent theoretical considerations (Crothers and Metzger, 1972) and experimental observations (reviewed by Hornick and Karush, 1972) have confirmed the validity of this early prediction concerning the advantage of multivalence in energetic terms, to the immune system.

The study of viral neutralization has provided much information relevant to the role of antibody multivalence in biological systems and there are several reports which show the reduction in neutralization of both animal viruses (Lafferty, 1963; Vogt *et al.*, 1964; Keller, 1966) and bacteriophages (Goodman and Donch, 1964; Klinman *et al.*, 1967; Stemke, 1969) when univalent antibodies have been used. However, a significant advance in this type of study was provided by the observation by Mäkelä (1966) that hapten-conjugated bacteriophage can be neutralized by anti-hapten antibody. Using 3-iodo-4-hydroxy-5-nitrophenyl acetyl (NIP)-conjugated T2 bacteriophage, Sarvas and Mäkelä (1970) obtained evidence for the superiority of IgM over IgG anti-NIP antibodies in neutralizing the phage and ascribed this superiority to the polyvalence of IgM. Hornick and Karush (1972) in a study of the neutralization of DNP-conjugated bacteriophage

ϕx174 by anti-DNP antibody have provided convincing evidence for the energetic advantage of polyvalent over monovalent antibody interaction with this polyvalent antigen. In these studies, IgG anti-DNP antibodies wish intrinsic affinity for the DNP group of 10^7 M^{-1} showed a functional affinity for DNP–ϕx174 of 10^{10} M^{-1}, which represents an enhancement due to divalent attachment of 1000-fold. In addition, degradation of IgG antibody to monovalent fragments resulted in a 100-fold reduction in functional affinity with no reduction in intrinsic affinity. On the other hand, IgM anti-DNP antibodies with an intrinsic affinity of 10^4–10^5 M^{-1} exhibited a functional affinity of 10^{11} M^{-1} which represents an enhancement due to multivalency of 10^6-fold. These authors suggest that this represents multivalent attachment of IgM–DNP to the conjugated phage *via* at least three of its binding sites.

Multivalent antibody binding has clear functional and biological advantages over monovalent binding. The most obvious advantage is the far lower concentration of multivalent antibody required for effective humoral immunity compared with the level of monovalent antibody which would be required for a similar degree of immunity.

Multivalence is of considerable importance in the binding of antigen by receptors on antigen-sensitive cells. Davie and Paul (1972a), and Bystryn *et al.* (1973) have demonstrated the enhanced binding of multivalent compared to monovalent ligands to cell-surface bound antibody. The latter authors showed that a multivalent DNP–conjugate bound to cells with an avidity which was 100–300-fold greater than that with a univalent DNP hapten. The high functional affinity of receptors on cells for multivalent antigens may render these interactions essentially irreversible, and viewed in the light of recent suggestions (Ramseier, 1971) that prolonged contact of antigen with antigen-sensitive cells is necessary for stimulation, points to an important role of polyvalent attachment in the initiation of the immune response. Evidence is available supporting a major assumption in the clonal selection theory (Burnet, 1959) that the affinity of cell receptors for antigen is the same as that of antibodies produced by progeny plasma cells (Siskind and Benacerraf, 1969; Mäkelä, 1970; Julius and Herzenberg, 1974). Cells with receptors of low intrinsic affinity for single antigenic determinants may, by virtue of polyvalent binding, bind antigen sufficiently well to be stimulated. Thus, the progeny of cells with receptors of high functional affinity—IgM—may produce low intrinsic affinity antibody. Polyvalent binding of antigen by cell-bound receptors may therefore be important in the production of low-affinity antibody and may explain why IgM antibodies often have lower K_0 values for hapten than IgG antibodies present in the serum at the same time (Mäkelä *et al.*, 1970).

In any discussion of the role of polyvalence in antibody affinity, the controversy concerning the valence of IgM must be considered (reviewed by Metzger, 1970). On the basis of its pentameric structure, it would be expected that IgM would exhibit decavalence for antigen. However, there are reports that IgM is pentavalent (Onoue *et al.*, 1965; Voss and Eisen, 1968), while there are others that the molecule is indeed decavalent (Cooper, 1967; Merler *et al.*, 1968;

Ashman and Metzger, 1969). Further controversy has been generated by the suggestion (Onoue *et al.*, 1968; Oriol and Rousset, 1974*a*, *b*) that there are five high and five low affinity antibody binding sites on a single molecule. However, Ashman and Metzger (1969) have suggested that an alternative explanation of the data of Onoue *et al.*, (1968) was the existence of heterogeneity among different molecules in the IgM population. It is clear that the valence of IgM is very much influenced by the size of the antigen used. Thus the observed valence of IgM anti-dextran antibody varied from 10 for dextran of molecular weight 342 to five for dextrans of molecular weights 7000–237 000; while with dextran of molecular weight of 1.87×10^6 the observed IgM antibody valence was 2·3 (Edberg *et al.*, 1972). Steric factors presumably play a role in the observations of reduced IgM valencies for certain antigens but cannot be invoked to explain reduced valencies for haptenic antigens.

6.2 Temporal Changes in Antibody Affinity

Progressive changes in the affinity or avidity of antibody with increasing time after immunization with a variety of antigens (toxins, viruses, or purified proteins) have been acknowledged for several years. Studies of the temporal changes in the affinity of antibodies to defined haptenic determinants (such as DNP) have confirmed the progressive increase in K_0 with time (Eisen and Siskind, 1964) and this phenomenon has been termed the 'maturation of the immune response' (Siskind and Benacerraf, 1969). That affinity maturation is the result of changes in the cell population producing antibody rather than the selective removal of high affinity antibody by the excess antigen present early in the response was demonstrated *in vitro* (Steiner and Eisen, 1967). The affinity of antibody produced *in vitro* by lymphoid cells taken from immunized rabbits early in the immune response is lower than that produced by cells taken late in the response.

Siskind and Benacerraf (1969) have expanded the clonal selection theory of Burnet (1959) to accommodate these observed variations in antibody affinity by suggesting that precursors of antibody-forming cells bind antigens *via* receptors having the same specificity and affinity as the antibody secreted by progeny cells. Thus, the maturation of the immune response is viewed as a progressive, antigen-driven preferential selection and stimulation of cells with the highest affinity receptors. Immunization with large doses of antigen in Freund's complete adjuvant results in a reduction in the rate of maturation of affinity compared to immunization with small doses (Eisen and Siskind, 1964), and this effect on affinity is consistent with this hypothesis and has been ascribed to the stimulation of even low affinity cells in the presence of excess antigen. Furthermore, under such situations it is possible that the high affinity cells may be rendered tolerant. Further evidence consistent with this hypothesis has been obtained at the serum level indicating progressive changes in the affinity distribution of antibody (Werblin and Siskind, 1972; Werblin *et al.*, 1973). If cells with high affinity receptors are indeed being selected preferentially by antigen, then during an

248

immune response these cells should be the most rapidly proliferating ones. Thus the use of cytotoxic drugs such as cyclophosphamide, which inhibit rapidly dividing cells, should preferentially inhibit high affinity antibody-producing cells, and antibody of low affinity would be produced. This indeed has been shown to be the case in groups of mice immunized with human serum albumin (HSA) in Freund's Complete Adjuvant and treated with increasing amounts of cyclophosphamide. In this case both levels and affinity of anti-HSA are reduced in treated compared to control mice. The levels and affinity of antibody decrease with increasing doses of cyclophosphamide (Steward *et al.*, 1973a).

The cell selection by antigen hypothesis also requires that the specificity and affinity of antigen receptors be correlated directly with the affinity and specificity of the antibody produced by progeny antibody-producing cells. Evidence consistent with this hypothesis has been obtained from recent studies in several laboratories (Andersson, 1970, 1972; Davie and Paul, 1972a, b, 1973; Claflin *et al.*, 1973; Claflin and Merchant, 1973; Julius and Herzenberg, 1974) in which

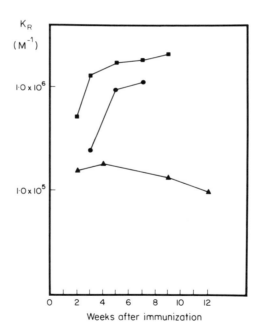

Figure 4 The effect of immunization of mice with human serum transferrin in Freund's complete adjuvant or with *Bordetella pertussis* on the increase in K_R with time compared to mice immunized with antigen in saline. ■, Freund's complete adjuvant; ●, *Bordetella pertussis*; ▲, saline. From Petty and Steward (1977a), reproduced by permission of Blackwell Scientific Publications Ltd

both the affinity of serum antibody and the avidity of antigen receptors on antigen-binding cells have been correlated with the avidity of antibody secreted at the plaque-forming cell level. There is clearly abundant evidence consistent with the concept of cell selection by antigen, resulting in a progressive increase in the affinity of serum antibody. However, observations of temporal changes in affinity, which cannot be interpreted readily on the basis of this concept, have been made. For example, Petty *et al.* (1972), Kimball (1972), and Urbain *et al.* (1972) have reported a fall in antibody affinity late in the immune response following the expected early rise.

The results of Petty *et al.* (1972) and Urbain *et al.* (1972) were obtained using mice and rabbits, respectively, which had been immunized with antigen in saline. The observations showing maturation of affinity with time and upon which the cell selection by antigen theory was based were obtained only following immunization in Freund's complete adjuvant. Mice showing a fall in affinity late in the immune response to antigen when injected in saline produce a long-lasting high-affinity response to the same antigen injected in Freund's complete and other adjuvants (Soothill and Steward, 1971; Petty and Steward, 1977*a*) (Figure 4). It is clear that the pattern of temporal changes in the affinity of serum antibody is affected markedly by the nature of the immunogenic stimulus. The antigen-depot effect produced by immunization in Freund's complete adjuvant with the resulting slow release of antigen over long periods results in sustained maturation of affinity. Immunization in saline results in the relatively rapid elimination of the antigen and subsequent termination of antigen stimulation. The fall in average affinity of serum antibody in this situation may be attributed to the death of short-lived high affinity antibody-producing cells. It is interesting to note that maturation of antibody affinity occurs with both Freund's complete adjuvant and *Bordetella pertussis* (see Figure 4). This observation suggests that affinity maturation is not restricted necessarily to adjuvants producing an antigen depot.

Other adjuvants, such as Freund's incomplete adjuvant, lipopolysaccharide B, BCG, alum precipitates, oestradiol, carbon, and latex also are able to enhance both level and affinity of anti-protein antibody. However, all these adjuvants vary in the degree to which they augment the parameters of the immune response. Some—Freund's complete and incomplete adjuvants, and carbon—induce the production of high levels of high affinity antibody, whereas the others elicit lower levels of high affinity antibody. The possibility therefore exists that adjuvants exert their influence on the antibody response at two stages: (*i*) at the level of antigen selection of cells for proliferation; and (*ii*) at the level of proliferation of antibody-forming cells (Petty and Steward, 1977*a*).

The observations of Kimball (1972) showing maturation and late fall in the affinity of antibody to type III pneumococcal antigen—which is not eliminated readily by mammals—indicate that competition for decreasing amounts of circulating antigen is not the only selective force for affinity maturation. Siskind *et al.* (1968) and Heller and Siskind (1973) have shown that passively administered antibody suppresses low affinity antibody-forming cells more readily than the high affinity cells, and results in an increase in the affinity of the antibody synthesized. It is, therefore, possible that the increase in affinity of anti-type III antibody is a consequence of the competition of antigen-sensitive cells and circulating antibody for antigen.

Other time-related variations in antibody affinity also have been reported in which there is an alteration of high and low affinity antibody during the immune response *in vivo* (Doria *et al.*, 1972; Kim and Karush, 1973) and *in vitro* (Macario and Conway de Macario, 1973). Furthermore, antibody responses have been described in which there is no demonstrable maturation of affinity during the immune response (Haber and Stone, 1969).

In view of the complex temporal changes in antibody affinity observed *in vivo* and *in vitro*, the concept of antigen-driven cell selection during the maturation of the immune response is perhaps an over-simplification. It has been suggested that there are at least four factors which are involved in the control of antibody affinity: (*i*) preferential selection of high affinity cells by antigen; (*ii*) tolerance induction in high affinity cells; (*iii*) the presence of circulating antibody; and (*iv*) the extent of cell proliferation during the response (Mond *et al.*, 1974).

6.3 Factors Affecting Antibody Affinity

In addition to the nature of the immunogenic stimulus, it is possible that several other variables determine the affinity of antibody in the circulation. These include genetic factors, reticuloendothelial system function, dietary factors, quantitative and qualitative aspects of lymphocyte function, and the effects of free antibody, antigen, or immune complexes.

6.3.1 Genetic Factors

The ability to respond to a range of natural and synthetic antigens by the production of specific immune responses is under autosomal-dominant genetic control and is, in many instances, associated with the histocompatibility antigens of the species concerned (McDevitt and Benacerraf, 1969; Benacerraf and McDevitt, 1972). Although strain-related variations in the specificity of antibodies to a variety of antigens in the mouse, guinea-pig, and rat have been demonstrated by several laboratories, conflicting evidence has been obtained by others. The existence of such variations in the affinity of antibody has only been reported by one laboratory using mice (Soothill and Steward, 1971; Petty *et al.*, 1972) and one using rats (Ruscetti *et al.*, 1974). The failure by many investigators to obtain evidence consistent with the genetic control of affinity may be due, in part, to the use of adjuvants in the immunization procedure (see p. 248–249).

Soothill and Steward (1971), and Petty *et al.* (1972) have demonstrated consistent strain-related differences in the affinity of antibodies produced in response to human serum albumin and human serum transferrin injected in saline (Figure 5). Similar, but less marked, differences were observed for antibody to the DNP hapten. Immunization with antigen Freund's complete adjuvant eliminates

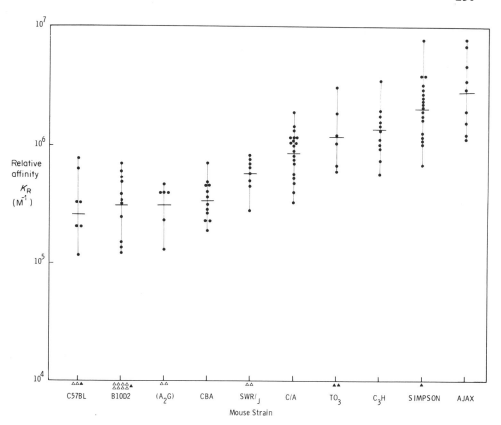

Figure 5 The relative affinity values K_R, of antibody to human serum albumin in 10 mouse strains. ▲, animals producing antibody but K_R values incalculable; △, animals not producing detectable antibody. From Petty *et al.*, 1972, reproduced by permission of Blackwell Scientific Publications Ltd.

these strain differences; all strains produce antibody of similar affinity of greater than 10^6 M^{-1}. Steward and Petty (1976) have measured the amount and affinity of antibody produced in response to protein antigens injected in saline in parents, F_1 hybrids, and backcross offspring of inbred mice that produce high ($>10^6$ M^{-1}) and low affinity ($<10^6$ M^{-1}) antibody to these antigens. The F_1 hybrids of the cross between a high-affinity strain (A/JAX) and a low-affinity strain (B10D 2 NEW) produced anti-human serum transferrin antibodies with a mean affinity between that of the two parents. When the F_1 hybrids were backcrossed to the high and low affinity parents, segregation of affinity values was observed which is consistent with some form of genetic control. Thus, the distribution of antibody affinity values in the (F_1 × high affinity parent) backcrosses are not significantly different from that of the high affinity parent strain. Similarly, the antibody produced by the (F_1 × low affinity parent) backcross have a distribution similar to the low affinity parents (Figure 6a).

252

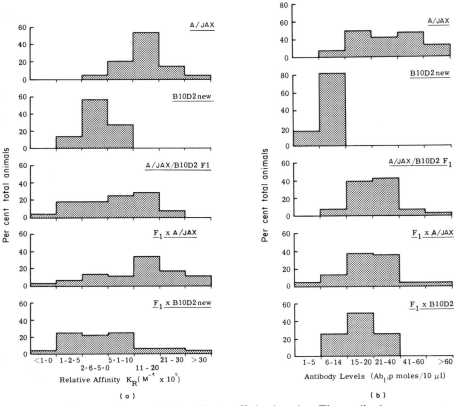

Figure 6 The genetic control of antibody affinity in mice. The antibody response to human serum transferrin in A/JAX and B10D2 new line mice, their F_1 hybrids, and backcross offspring. (a) Relative affinity K_R of antibody, and (b) antibody levels, Ab_t. From Steward and Petty (1976), reproduced by permission of Blackwell Scientific Publications Ltd.

Antibody levels, however, do not show the same trend as that observed for affinity (Figure 6b) and are not correlated with affinity. The results confirm the suggestion of genetic control of antibody affinity indicated in Figure 5, and furthermore indicate that antibody levels and affinity are two parameters of the immune response which are under independent genetic control.

Ruscetti *et al.* (1974) have reported that the affinity of antibodies to poly (Glu$_{52}$, Lys$_{33}$, Tyr$_{15}$) injected in Freund's complete adjuvant into rats is under genetic control. These workers demonstrated that high-responding strains produce higher affinity antibody than do the low-responding strains. They also reported that the use of aggregated antigen increases both the level and affinity of antibody in the low-responder strains, but decreased both parameters in the high-responding ones. These data thus underline the importance of the nature of the immunogenic stimulus in the affinity of antibody.

Further evidence confirming the genetic control of antibody affinity has been obtained by Katz and Steward (1975). Mice from an initial random-bred

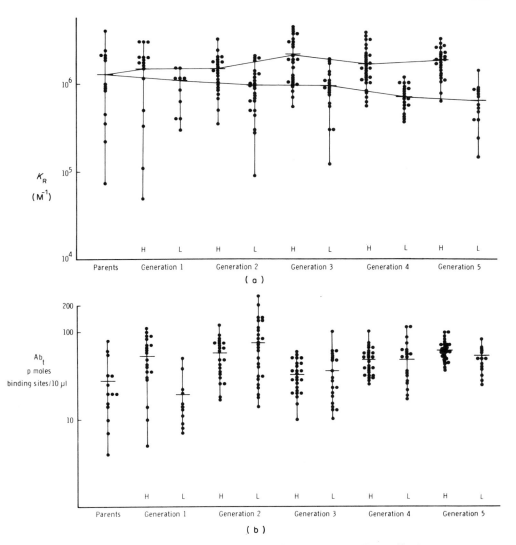

Figure 7 The genetic control of antibody affinity in mice. The antibody response to protein antigens in TO mice selectively bred on the basis of antibody affinity (K_R) into two lines; H, high affinity line; L, low affinity line. (a) Relative affinity values, K_R; and (b) antibody levels, Ab_t. After Katz and Steward (1975)

population were bred selectively on the basis of the affinity the antibody produced to protein antigens injected in saline. At each generation of selective breeding, mice producing antibody (with affinity greater than 10^6 M^{-1}) were mated. Similarly mice producing antibody with affinity lower than 10^6 M^{-1} were mated. After five generations of selective breeding, differences on affinity between the two lines were highly significant ($p < 0.0005$), whereas antibody levels were not significantly different ($p < 0.2$). This breeding programme has resulted in a progressive separation of the two lines with regard to antibody affinity, but has not produced a corresponding separation of antibody levels (Figure 7a, b). These results suggest that antibody affinity is under polygenic control and that it is exerted independently of that controlling antibody levels.

6.3.2 The Role of the Reticuloendothelial System

It is clear that macrophages play an important part in the afferent limb of the immune response. Transfer experiments have demonstrated that macrophages co-operate with T and B lymphocytes in initiating and achieving an optimal antibody response (Unanue and Cerrottini, 1970; Feldman, 1972), and antigen that has been processed by macrophages shows increased immunogenicity compared to the unprocessed antigen (Unanue, 1972). Furthermore, the use of agents affecting macrophage function, such as adjuvants (Spitznagel and Allison, 1970) and carbon (Sabet et al., 1969; Souhami, 1972) can either enhance or decrease antibody titres. In view of this central role of macrophages in the immune response, the possibility exists that differences in macrophage function could result in variations in antibody affinity as well as in antibody levels. This suggestion is supported by the observation that adjuvants increase both levels and affinity of antibody in inbred strains of mice (Soothill and Steward, 1971), whereas blockade of macrophages by carbon reduces antibody affinity but does not alter antibody levels (Passwell et al., 1974a). Inbred strains of mice differ in the affinity of antibody they produce to antigens injected in saline (see Figure 5). Using the clearance of colloidal carbon as a measure of macrophage function, Passwell et al. (1974a) have shown that the production of low affinity antibody corresponds to either poor carbon clearance or slow recovery from carbon blockade. However, Morgan and Soothill (1975) have utilized the clearance of $[^{125}I]$ polyvinyl pyrolidone as a measure of macrophage function and have demonstrated a more precise correlation between antibody affinity and macrophage function. The ranking orders of of the mouse strains for both K_{PVP} (the constant for the clearance of PVP) and for K_R (antibody affinity) correlate significantly. These authors suggested that the more precise correlation of PVP clearance with affinity compared to that of carbon clearance with affinity may be because PVP is more similar in size to immunogenic microaggregates of soluble proteins than the carbon particles are, and that partial macrophage blockade may have occurred with the dose of carbon used.

These in vivo correlations of macrophage function with antibody affinity have been confirmed recently by in vitro experiments. The uptake of radiolabelled immune complexes by cultured peritoneal macrophages from several inbred mouse strains have been found to correlate with the affinity of serum antibody (Wiener and Steward, unpublished data).

The importance of macrophage function in determining the affinity of antibody is further supported by the observations that other factors affecting macrophage activity also result in a corresponding effect on antibody affinity. (i)

Oestrogens, which stimulate macrophage function (Flemming, 1967), produce an increased carbon clearance and high-affinity production in mice normally producing low affinity antibody (Passwell *et al.*, 1974*a*). (*ii*) Protein deprivation suppresses macrophage function and results in the production of low affinity antibody in mice normally producing high affinity (Passwell *et al.*, 1974*b*). (*iii*) Infection with malaria leads to macrophage blockade, and mice normally producing high affinity antibody synthesize low affinity antibody following the infection (Steward and Voller, 1973).

The observations cited here serve to illustrate the possible role of macrophages in determining the affinity of serum antibody. The precise way in which 'poor' macrophage function leads to low affinity antibody synthesis and 'good' macrophage function to high affinity antibody production is not known. However, it is possible that poor function leads to inefficient processing of antigen and presentation to immunocompetent cells. Spitznagel and Allison (1970) have suggested that macrophages prevent tolerance by limiting the access of antigen to B cells. The possibility, therefore, exists that in animals with poor macrophage function, antigen (perhaps 'unprocessed') reaches the B cells and preferentially induces tolerance in high affinity cells which are more susceptible to this induction (Theis and Siskind, 1968). Data in support of this hypothesis have been obtained from experiments with mouse strains producing either high or low affinity antibody when injected with antigen in saline (Steward *et al.*, 1974). 'High affinity' and 'low affinity' mice were preimmunized with antigen in saline and then challenged with antigen in Freund's complete adjuvant. Both preimmunized and non-preimmunized high affinity mice produced high affinity antibody on challenge. However, preimmunized low affinity mice produced low affinity antibody on challenge, whereas non-preimmunized low affinity mice produced the high affinity antibody. These results suggest that the preimmunization of low affinity mice results in some form of immunological tolerance—because of a possible macrophage defect—in which high affinity cells are unable to respond to the challenge of antigen in adjuvant.

6.3.3 Other Factors

It is very probable that several other factors affect the affinity of antibody produced by an animal. It is particularly likely that qualitative and quantitative variations in lymphocyte function play an important role in this regard. Indeed, Gershon and Paul (1971) have shown that T cells are required for the production of high-affinity anti-hapten antibody and that the affinity of the antibody produced is in part determined by the number of T cells present in the immunized animal. However, Taniguchi and Tada (1974) have obtained contradictory evidence showing the augmentation of antibody affinity in rabbits following thymectomy of adults. This observation was confirmed and extended in mice by Takemori and Tada (1974), who demonstrated that adoptive transfer of thymus or spleen cells from carrier-primed donors results in a significant decrease in the avidity of anti-DNP plaque-forming cell antibodies (in both primary and secondary responses) produced by syngeneic recipients following immunization with DNP–carrier.

The New Zealand mice show a progressive loss in T-cell helper function with age (Denman and Denman, 1970), and a similar age-related loss of suppressor function precedes the loss of helper function (Gerber *et al.*, 1974). It is therefore possible that the fall in affinity of anti-protein antibody with increasing age (Petty and Steward, 1977*b*) may be related to the loss of T cells. A similar fall in the avidity of antibody to DNA in NZB/W F_1 hybrid mice with increasing age (Steward *et al.*, 1975) may also be a result of T-cell deficiencies. Furthermore, these mice show a progressive fall in macrophage function as assessed by PVP clearance (Morgan and Steward, 1976). This fall in macrophage function with increasing age may be an age-related defect in the macrophages themselves or alternatively may be a consequence of reticuloendothial system fatigue arising from the excess of circulating DNA–anti-DNA complexes in these mice. In older mice, the affinity of antibody therefore may be affected as a result of impaired antigen processing by the fatigued reticuloendothelial system. The fall in the avidity of circulating anti-DNA antibody in NZB/W F_1 hybrid mice may arise from yet another factor which affects antibody affinity—circulating antigen. In the presence of excess circulating antigen, high affinity antibody may be removed in a complexed form leaving predominantly low affinity antibody in the circulation. This argument also applies to any situation in which antigen is likely to be present in excess. Rheumatoid factors have been shown to be of low affinity (Normansell, 1970; Steward *et al.*, 1975), but since the corresponding antigen (autologous IgG) is present in excess, the low affinity serum antibody may be that remaining after elimination of the high affinity antibody in immune complex form.

A further factor that may affect the affinity of antibody produced is circulating antibody. Such antibody may compete with antigen-sensitive cells for antigen and increase the affinity of the antibody subsequently produced. Furthermore, it has been shown that low affinity antibody-forming cells are suppressed more readily by passively transferred antibody than are high affinity cells, and that low affinity is less efficient at such suppression than is high affinity antibody (Siskind *et al.*, 1968; Walker and Siskind, 1969). Finally, Werblin *et al.* (1973) have shown that in a genetically diverse population of rabbits, the a1 allotype is associated with the production of high affinity antibody and the a6 allotype with low affinity antibody to the DNP hapten. These observations therefore suggest that structural variations in the V_H region of the molecule may influence antibody affinity.

6.4 The Biological and Immunopathological Significance of Antibody Affinity

Since experimental evidence supports the concept of a progressive selection of cells capable of producing the highest affinity antibody and that antibody multivalence provides an enormous amplification in energetic terms in the antibody–antigen reaction, it would seem that it is biologically important for an

Table 4 Biological reactions in which high affinity antibody is more effective than low affinity antibody

Reaction	Reference
Destruction of D-positive erythrocytes	Hughes-Jones (1967)
Passive haemagglutination	Levine and Levytska (1967)
Complement fixation	Fauci *et al.* (1970)
	Warner and Ovary (1970)
Passive cutaneous anaphylaxis	Fauci *et al.* (1970)
	Warner and Ovary (1970)
Haemolysis	Warner and Ovary (1970)
Immune elimination	Alpers *et al.* (1972)
Virus neutralization	Blank *et al.* (1972)
Membrane damage	Six *et al.* (1973)
Enzyme inactivation	Erickson (1974)
Protective capacity against bacteria	Ahlstedt *et al.* (1974)

animal to develop high affinity antibody in response to an immunological challenge. Furthermore, data are available which demonstrate the superiority of high affinity compared with low affinity antibodies in biological reactions, including several which are of importance in providing effective immunity in the host. Some of the biological reactions in which high affinity antibody is more effective are listed in Table 4.

Aside from the perhaps obvious advantage of high affinity antibody in forming potentially more stable bonds with antigen, the superiority of high affinity antibody in reactions such as complement fixation, may arise from the more efficient induction of essential conformational changes in the antibody molecule occurring as a result of high affinity reactions with the antigen. The evidence for conformational changes in antibody structure following interaction with antigen is discussed elsewhere in this volume (see Feinstein, Chapter 8).

When reading the literature on the subject of antibody affinity, one can gain the impression that the role of low affinity antibody in the immune response is merely as an intermediate in the pathway towards high affinity antibody production, and that cells producing the former are eliminated somehow during affinity maturation. However, recent work by, for example, Werblin and Siskind (1972) has illustrated that low affinity antibodies persist throughout the immune response, even though they are perhaps of secondary importance to high affinity antibodies. The possibility exists that, since cells with low affinity receptors are less readily susceptible to tolerance induction by antigen than cells with high affinity receptors (Theis and Siskind, 1968), the persistence of low affinity cells may provide a useful first-line defence against antigenic insult by the production of antibody (particularly IgM) having low intrinsic affinity but high functional affinity (or avidity). It is possible that low affinity antibody may also be of value in amplifying complement-fixation reactions by binding first to one site on a cell membrane, fixing complement, and, then because of its low affinity, dissociating from the first site, thus becoming free to bind a second site and to activate the complement system again.

Quite apart from the difficulty in adequately assigning a positive role to low-affinity antibody, there has been interest in the possibility that a predominantly low affinity antibody response may be viewed as an expression of immuno-deficiency (Soothill and Steward, 1971 *et al.*, 1972). As discussed in Section 6.3, the affinity of an antibody response can be influenced by a variety of factors including genetic and environmental ones, abnormalities in macrophage and T-cell helper function, and other lymphocyte abnormalities such as increased susceptibility to tolerance induction of high affinity antigen-sensitive cells (Steward *et al.*, 1974). Such a genetically determined low affinity antibody response to viral or microbial infections may have serious immunopathological consequences in the host as the antibody would be likely to fail to eliminate the antigen (Alpers *et al.*, 1972), thus favouring the production and persistence of antigen-excess immune complexes in the circulation. These complexes could either be formed with the low affinity antibody itself or with any high affinity antibody produced by the host; complement-mediated damage would follow their subsequent deposition in tissues. This hypothesis is being investigated currently in both human and murine immune complex diseases (Steward, 1976) and is outlined schematically in Figure 8.

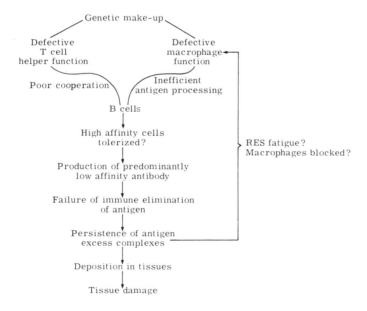

Figure 8 Schematic representation of the possible role of low affinity antibody in immune complex disease. From Steward (1976), reproduced by permission of Blackwell Scientific Publications Ltd.

ACKNOWLEDGEMENTS

Work in the author's laboratory cited here was aided by a grant from the Medical Research Council. Financial support from the Arthritis and Rheumatism Council also is acknowledged gratefully.

The author thanks Miss J. S. Linfield for help in the preparation of the manuscript.

REFERENCES

Ahlstedt, S., Holmgren, J., and Hanson, L. A. (1973. *Immunology*, **25**, 917.
Ahlstedt, S., Holmgren, J., and Hanson, L. A. (1974). *Int. Archs. Allergy appl. Immunol.*, **46**, 470.
Alpers, J. H., Steward, M. W., and Soothill, J. F. (1972). *Clin. Exp. Immunol.*, **12**, 21.
Andersson, B. (1970). *J. Exp. Med.*, **132**, 77.
Andersson, B. (1972). *J. Exp. Med.*, **135**, 312.
Ashman, R. F., and Metzger, H. (1969). *J. Biol. Chem.*, **244**, 3405

Barisas, B. G., Singer, S. J., and Sturtevant, J. M. (1975. *Immunochemistry*, **12**, 411.
Benacerraf, B., and McDevitt, H. O. (1972). *Science, N.Y.*, **175**, 273.
Blank, S. E., Leslie, G. A., and Clem, L. W. (1972). *J. Immunol.*, **108**, 665.
Burnet, F. M. (1959). *The Clonal Selection Theory of Acquired Immunity*, Cambridge University Press, Cambridge.
Burnet, F. M., Keogh, E. V., and Lush, D. (1937). *Aust. J. Exp. Biol. Med. Sci.*, **15**, 226.
Bystryn, J. C., Siskind, G. W., and Uhr, J. W. (1973). *J. Exp. Med.*, **137**, 301.

Celada, F., Schmidt, D., and Strom, R. (1969). *Immunology*, **17**, 189.
Chance, B. (1963). In *Technique of Organic Chemistry* Vol. 8, part II, Interscience, New York.
Claflin, L., Merchant, B., and Inman, J. (1973). *J. Immunol.*, **110**, 241.
Claflin, L., and Merchant, B. (1973). *J. Immunol.*, **110**, 252.
Cooper, A. G. (1967). *Science, N.Y.*, **157**, 933.
Crothers, D. M., and Metzger, U. (1972). *Immunochemistry*, **9**, 341.

Dandliker, W. B., Schapio, H. C., Meduski, J. W., Alonso, R., Feigen, G. A., and Hamrick, J. R., Jr. (1964). *Immunochemistry*, **1**, 165.
Davie, J. M., and Paul, W. E. (1972a). *J. Exp. Med.*, **135**, 643.
Davie, J. M., and Paul, W. E. (1972b). *J. Exp. Med.*, **135**, 660.
Davie, J. M., and Paul, W. E. (1973). *J. Exp. Med.*, **137**, 201.
Day, E. D. (1972). *Advanced Immunochemistry*, Williams and Wilkins, Baltimore, p. 181.
Day, L. A., Sturtevant, J. M., and Singer, S. T. (1963). *Ann. N.Y. Acad. Sci.*, **103**, 611.
Denman, A. M., and Denman, E. J. (1970). *Clin. Exp. Immunol.*, **6**, 457.
Doria, G., Schiaffini, G., Garavini, M., and Mancini, C. (1972). *J. Immunol.*, **109**, 1245.

Edberg, D., Bronson, P., and Van Oss, C. J. (1972). *Immunochemistry*, **9**, 273.
Eigen, M., and DeMaeyer, L. (1963). In *Techniques of Organic Chemistry* Vol. 8, part II, Interscience, New York.
Eisen, H. N. (1964). *Methods Med. Res.*, **10**, 106.
Eisen, H. N., and Siskind, G. W. (1964). *Biochemistry*, **3**, 996.
Erickson, R. P. (1974). *Immunochemistry*, **11**, 41.

Farr, R. S. (1958). *J. infect. Dis.*, **103**, 239.

260

Fauci, A. S., Frank, M. M., and Johnson, J. S. (1970). *J. Immunol.*, **105**, 215.
Fazekas de St. Groth, S. (1961). *Aust. J. Exp. Biol. Med. Sci.*, **39**, 563.
Feldman, M. (1972). *J. Exp. Med.*, **135**, 1049.
Ferber, J. M. (1965). M.S. Thesis, MIT, Cambridge, Mass.
Fleming, K. B. P. (1967). *Adv. Exp. Med. Biol.*, **1**, 188.
Froese, A. (1968). *Immunochemistry*, **5**, 253.
Froese, A., and Sehon, A. H. (1965). *Immunochemistry*, **2**, 135.
Froese, A. and Sehon, A. H. (1971). In *Methods in Immunology and Immunochemistry*,
   Vol. III, (Chase, M., and Williams, C., Eds) Academic Press, New York and London,
   p. 412.
Froese, A., and Sehon, A. H. (1975). *Contemp. Top. Mol. Immunol.*, **4**, p. 23.
Froese, A., Sehon, A. H., and Eigen, M. (1962). *Can. J. Chem.*, **40**, 1786.

Gaze S. E., West, N. J., and Steward, M. W. (1973). *J. Immunol. Methods*, **3**, 357.
Gerber, N. L., Hardin, J. A., Chused, T. M., and Steinberg, A. D. (1974). *J. Immunol.*, **113**,
   1618.
Gershon, R. K., and Paul, W. E. (1971). *J. Immunol.*, **106**, 872.
Goldberg, R. J., and Campbell, D. M. (1951). *J. Immunol.*, **66**, 79.
Goodman, J. W., and Donch, J. J. (1964). *J. Immunol.*, **93**, 96.

Haber, E., and Stone, M. (1969). *Israel J. Med. Sci.*, **5**, 332.
Haselkorn, D., Pecht, I., Friedman, S., Yaron, A., Givol, D., and Sela, M. (1971). *Israel J.
   Chem.*, **9**, 53.
Haustein, D. (1971). Doctoral Dissertation, Universitat Freiberg, Germany.
Heidelberger, M., and Kendall, F. E. (1935). *J. Exp. Med.*, **61**, 563.
Heller, K. S., and Siskind, G. W. (1973). *Cell. Immunol.*, **6**, 59.
Herbert, V., Lau, K. S., Gottleib, C. W., and Bleicher, S. J. J. (1965). *Clin. Endocrinol.
   Metab.*, **25**, 1375.
Hooker, S. B., and Boyd, W. C. (1935). *J. Gen. Physiol.*, **19**, 373.
Hornick, C. L., and Karush, F. (1972). *Immunochemistry*, **9**, 325.
Hughes-Jones, N. C. (1967). *Immunology*, **12**, 565.

Julius, M. H., and Herzenberg, L. A. (1974). *J. Exp. Med.*, **140**, 904.

Karush, F. (1956). *J. Am. Chem. Soc.*, **78**, 5519.
Karush, F. (1962). *Adv. Immunol.*, **2**, 1.
Karush, F. (1970). *Ann. N.Y. Acad. Sci.*, **169**, 56.
Katz, F. E., and Steward, M. W. (1975). *Immunology*, **29**, 543.
Keller, R. (1966). *J. Immunol.*, **96**, 96.
Kelly, K. A., Sehon, A. H., and Froese, A. (1971). *Immunochemistry*, **8**, 613.
Kim, Y. D., and Karush, F. (1973). *Immunochemistry*, **10**, 365.
Kimball, J. W. (1972). *Immunochemistry*, **9**, 1169.
Klinman, N. R., Long, C., and Karush, F. (1967). *J. Immunol.*, **99**, 1128.

Lafferty, K. J. (1963). *Virology*, **21**, 61.
Levine, B. B., and Levytska, V. (1967). *J. Immunol.*, **98**, 648.
Levison, S. A., Portman, A. J., Kierszenbaum, F., and Dandliker, W. B. (1971). *Biochem.
   Biophys. Res. Commun.*, **43**, 258.

Macario, A. J. L., and Conway de Macario, E. (1973). *Nature, (Lond.)*, **245**, 263.
Mäkelä, O. (1966). *Immunology*, **10**, 81.
Mäkelä, O. (1970). *Transplant. Rev.*, **5**, 3.
Mäkelä, O., Ruoslahati, E., and Seppälä, I. J. T. (1970). *Immunochemistry*, **7**, 917.

McDevitt, H. O., and Benacerraf, B. (1969). *Adv. Immunol.*, **11**, 31.
Medof, M. E., and Aladjem, F. (1971). *Fed. Proc.*, **30**, 657.
Merler, E., Karlin, L., and Matsumoto, S. (1968). *J. Biol. Chem.*, **243**, 386.
Metzger, H. (1970). *Adv. Immunol.*, **12**, 57.
Mond, J., Kim, Y. T., and Siskind, G. W. (1974). *J. Immunol.*, **112**, 1255.
Morgan, A. G., and Soothill, J. F. (1975). *Nature (Lond.)*, **254**, 711.
Morgan, A. G., and Steward, M. W. (1976). *Clin. Exp. Immunol.*, **26**, 133.
Mukkur, T. K. S., Szewczuk, M. R., and Schmidt, D. E., Jr. (1974). *Immunochemistry*, **11**, 9.

Nisonoff, A., and Pressman, D. (1958). *J. Immunol.*, **80**, 417.
Normansell, D. E. (1970). *Immunochemistry*, **7**, 787.

Onoue, K., Yagi, Y., Grossberg, A. L., and Pressman, D. (1965). *Immunochemistry*, **2**, 401.
Onoue, K., Yagi, Y., Grossberg, A. L., and Pressman, D. (1968). *Science, N.Y.*, **162**, 574.
Oriol, R., and Rousset, M. (1974*a*). *J. Immunol.*, **112**, 2227.
Oriol, R., and Rousset, M. (1974*b*). *J. Immunol.*, **112**, 2235.

Parker, C. W., Yoo, T. J., Johnson, M. C., and Godt, S. M. (1967). *Biochemistry*, **6**, 3408.
Passwell, J. H., Steward, M. W., and Soothill, J. F. (1974*a*). *Clin. Exp. Immunol.*, **17**, 159.
Passwell, J. H., Steward, M. W., and Soothill, J. F. (1974*b*). *Clin. Exp. Immunol.*, **17**, 491.
Paul, W. E., and Elfenbein, G. J. (1975). *J. Immunol.*, **114**, 261.
Pauling, L., Pressman, D., and Grossberg, A. L. (1944). *J. Am. Chem. Soc.*, **66**, 784.
Pecht, I., Givol, D., and Sela, M. (1972*a*). *J. Mol. Biol.*, **68**, 241.
Pecht, I., Haselkorn, D., and Friedman, S. (1972*b*). *FEBS Letters*, **24**, 331.
Petty, R. E., and Steward, M. W. (1977*a*). *Immunology*, **32**, 49.
Petty, R. E., and Steward, M. W. (1977*b*). *Ann. Rheumat. Dis.*, **36**, 39.
Petty, R. E., Steward, M. W., and Soothill, J. F. (1972). *Clin. Exp. Immunol.*, **12**, 231.
Pressman, D., Roholt, O. A., and Grossberg, A. L. (1970). *Ann. N.Y. Acad. Sci.*, **169**, 65.
Ramseier, H. (1971). *Eur. J. Immunol.*, **1**, 171.
Ruscetti, S. K., Kunz, H. W., and Gill, T. J. (1974). *J. Immunol.*, **113**, 1468.

Sabet, T., Newlin, L., and Friedman, H. (1969). *Immunology*, **16**, 433.
Sarvas, H., and Mäkelä, O. (1970). *Immunochemistry*, **7**, 933.
Scatchard, G. (1949). *Ann. N.Y. Acad. Sci.*, **51**, 660.
Schirrmacher, V. (1972). *Eur. J. Immunol.*, **2**, 430.
Sips, R. (1948). *J. Chem. Phys.*, **16**, 490.
Siskind, G. W., and Benacerraf, B. (1969). *Adv. Immunol.*, **10**, 1.
Siskind, G. W., Dunn, P., and Walker, J. G. (1968). *J. Exp. Med.*, **127**, 55.
Six, H. R., Uemura, K., and Kinsky, S. C. (1973). *Biochemistry*, **12**, 4003.
Skubitz, K. M., and Smith, T. W. (1975). *J. Immunol.*, **114**, 1369.
Smith, T. W., and Skubitz, K. M. (1975). *Biochemistry*, **14**, 1496.
Soothill, J. F., and Steward, M. W. (1971). *Clin. Exp. Immunol.*, **9**, 193.
Souhami, R. L. (1972). *Immunology*, **22**, 685.
Spitznagel, J. K., and Allison, A. C. (1970). *J. Immunol.*, **104**, 128.
Steiner, L. A., and Eisen, H. N. (1967). *J. Exp. Med.*, **126**, 1161.
Stemke, E. W. (1969). *J. Immunol.*, **103**, 596.
Steward, M. W. (1976). In *Infection and Immunology in the Rheumatic Diseases* (Dumonde, D. C., ed.), Blackwell, Oxford, p. 439.
Steward, M. W., Alpers, J. H., and Soothill, J. F. (1973*a*). *Proc. Roy. Soc. Med.*, **66**, 808.
Steward, M. W., Gaze, S. E., and Petty, R. E. (1974). *Eur. J. Immunol.*, **4**, 751.
Steward, M. W., Katz, F. E., and West, N. J. (1975). *Clin. Exp. Immunol.*, **21**, 121.
Steward, M. W., and Petty, R. E. (1972*a*). *Immunology*, **23**, 881.

Steward, M. W., and Petty, R. E. (1972*b*). *Immunology*, **22**, 747.

Steward, M. W., and Petty, R. E. (1976). *Immunology*, **30**, 789.

Steward, M. W., Turner, M. W., Natvig, J. B., and Gaarder, P. I. (1973*b*). *Clin. Exp. Immunol.*, **15**, 145.

Steward, M. W., and Voller, A. (1973). *Brit. J. Exp. Pathol.*, **54**, 198.

Stupp, V., Yoshida, T., and Paul, W. E. (1969). *J. Immunol.*, **103**, 625.

Takemori, T., and Tada, T. (1974). *J. Exp. Med.*, **140**, 253.

Taliaferro, W. H., Taliaferro, L. G., and Pizzi, A. K. (1959). *J. Infect. Dis.*, **105**, 197.

Taniguchi, M., and Tada, T. (1974). *J. Exp. Med.*, **139**, 108.

Talmage, D. W. (1960). *J. Infect. Dis.*, **107**, 115.

Taylor, R. B. (1975). *Immunology*, **29**, 989.

Theis, G. A., and Siskind, G. W. (1968). *J. Immunol.*, **100**, 138.

Unanue, E. R. (1972). *Adv. Immunol.*, **15**, 95.

Unanue, E. R., and Cerrottini, J. C. (1970). *Semin. Hematol.*, **7**, 225.

Urbain, J., van Acker, A., De Vos-Cloetens, C. H., and Urbain-Vansanten, G. (1972). *Immunochemistry*, **9**, 121.

Velick, S. F., Parker, C. W., and Eisen, H. N. (1960). *Proc. Nat. Acad. Sci., U.S.A.*, **46**, 1470.

Vogt, A., Kopp, R., Mass, G., and Reich, L. (1964). *Science, N.Y.*, **145**, 144.

Voss, E. W., and Eisen, H. N. (1968) *Fed. Proc.*, **27**, 2361.

Walker, J. G., and Siskind, G. W. (1969). *J. Exp. Med.*, **127**, 55.

Warner, N. L., and Ovary, Z. (1970). *J. Immunol.*, **105**, 812.

Werblin, T. P., Kim, Y. T., Mage, R., Benacerraf, B., and Siskind, G. W. (1973). *Immunology*, **25**, 17.

Werblin, T. P., and Siskind, G. W. (1972). *Immunochemistry*, **9**, 987.

CHAPTER 8

Models of Immunoglobulins and Antigen–Antibody Complexes

A. Feinstein and D. Beale

1 INTRODUCTION

In this chapter an account will be given of the structural background needed for the consideration of changes that might take place in antibodies when they bind to antigen.

The recognition of amino acid sequence homology regions in the polypeptide chains of IgG (Hill *et al.*, 1967; Edelman *et al.*, 1969) led to the development of the domain hypothesis (Edelman and Gall, 1969). This hypothesis postulated that each immunoglobulin chain is folded into several globular regions with different biological functions.

Several groups of X-ray crystallographers have confirmed the domain hypothesis; their work has been reviewed by Poljak (1975*a, b*) and by Davies *et al.* (1975*a, b*). It has become possible to speculate on the biological functions of

263

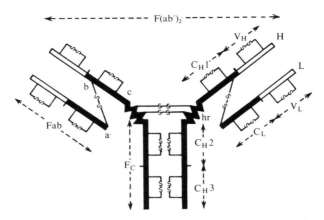

Figure 1 Chemical structure of human IgG4. L, light chain; H, heavy chain; hr, extra-domain hinge region; and –S–S–, cystine disulphide bridge. Light and heavy chains are represented as extended structures by lines, which are shaded for C regions and unshaded for V regions. Each chain has been divided into domains and each domain has an intra-chain disulphide bridge. Fab, F(ab')$_2$, and Fc indicate proteolytic fragments

immunoglobulins in three-dimensional terms and such an approach has been made by Beale and Feinstein (1976).

2 BASIC IMMUNOGLOBULIN STRUCTURE

Numerous laboratories, but particularly those of Porter and of Edelman, contributed to the early studies of immunoglobulin structure. This work has been reviewed extensively by Cohen and Porter (1964), Cohen and Milstein (1967) and Turner in Chapter I of this book. In addition, Porter (1973) has given a general account of the structure of immunoglobulins, hence only a brief outline will be included in this chapter.

Immunoglobulins can be regarded as being based on a common structure of two light and two heavy polypeptide chains linked by the disulphide bridges of cystine residues. The structure of human IgG4 is shown in Figure 1. Light chains

Table 1 Polypeptide chain composition of immunoglobulins

Immunoglobulin	Polypeptide chains
IgG1	$(L-\gamma_1)_2$
IgG4	$(L-\gamma_4)_2$
IgM	$[(L-\mu)_2]_5 J$
IgA	$(L-\alpha)_2$ or $[(L-\alpha)_2]_2 J$
IgE	$(L-\varepsilon)_2$
IgD	$(L-\delta)_2$

occur as two types (κ or λ) and are common to all normal immunoglobulins. They consist of a domain (V_L) of variable amino acid sequence, involved in antigen binding, and a domain (C_L) of constant amino acid sequence. Each domain has an essential intra-chain disulphide bridge. Heavy chains of different primary structure determine the class and subclass of immunoglobulins (Table 1). Different classes of H chain differ in their number of domains and non-domain regions. These variations are summarized in Table 2.

Table 2 Domain composition of immuno-globulin chains

Chain	Composition				
Light chain					
λ	V_λ	C_λ			
κ	V_κ	C_κ			
Heavy chain					
γ	V_H	$C_\gamma 1$	hr	$C_\gamma 2$	$C_\gamma 3$
μ	V_H	$C_\mu 1$	$C_\mu 3$	$C_\mu 3$	$C_\mu 4$ tp
α	V_H	$C_\alpha 1$	hr	$C_\alpha 2$	$C_\alpha 3$ tp
ε	V_H	$C_\varepsilon 1$	$C_\varepsilon 2$	$C_\varepsilon 3$	$C_\varepsilon 4$

hr, hinge region; tp, tail piece

Amino acid sequence studies of IgG predicted that the γ chain has four domains (V_γ, $C_\gamma 1$, $C_\gamma 2$, $C_\gamma 3$) (Edelman *et al.*, 1969) with a short 'hinge' region lying between the $C_\gamma 1$ and $C_\gamma 2$ domains (see Figure 1). It is within this region that flexibility between the two Fab units and Fc occurs.

In human and mouse IgG1 the light-heavy disulphide bridge joins a to c rather than a to b in IgG4 (Figure 1). In rabbit IgG there is an additional intra-chain bridge joining b to c. Due to the three-dimensional folding of a domain (see Figure 4) a, b, and c are really close together in space. The hinge region differs in the number of residues and disulphide bridges depending on the species and subclass of IgG. Fab and Fc fragments are produced by proteolytic cleavage between the C_H1 domain and the hinge region. F(ab')$_2$ fragment is formed by cleavage between the hinge region and C_H2 domain. IgG3 and IgA have extended hinge regions. IgA has an extra-domain tail piece immediately following the C_H3 domain. IgA can form dimers and tetramers.

Similar studies of IgM indicate that the μ chain has five domains (V_H, $C_\mu 1$, $C_\mu 2$, $C_\mu 3$, $C_\mu 4$) (Putnam *et al.*, 1973; Watanabe *et al.*, 1973) with an additional non-domain 'tail' piece of 19 residues immediately following the $C_\mu 4$ domain (Figure 2). J Chain is found linked by disulphide bonds to the tail piece (Mestecky and Schrohenloher, 1974) and probably regulates intra-cellular polymerization (see reviews by Inman and Mestecky, 1975; Koshland, 1975; and Parkhouse, Chapter 3 of this volume). The μ chain has no sequence analogous to the hinge region of the γ chain. The genetic information for this region probably replaces that for a domain deleted from the ancestral gene. Thus, immunoglobulins have either a non-domain hinge region or an additional domain.

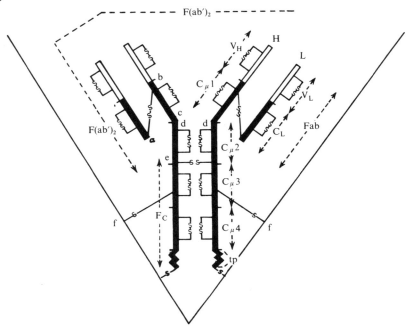

Figure 2   The human IgM 7S subunit. L, light chain; H, heavy chain (μ); tp, extra-domain tail piece; –S–S–, cystine disulphide bridge. In the cyclic 19 S molecule five subunits are disulphide bridged with a J chain. Fab fragment is formed by proteolytic cleavage between the $C_\mu 1$ and $C_\mu 2$ domains. $F(ab')_2$ is formed by cleavage just below, and $(Fc)_5$ just above, bridge e

Sequence studies on the α chain (Putnam, 1974; Kratzin *et al.*, 1975; Low *et al.*, 1976) have revealed the presence of four domains (V_H, $C_\alpha 1$, $C_\alpha 2$, $C_\alpha 3$). There is a non-domain region lying between the $C_\alpha 1$ and $C_\alpha 2$ domains which is analogous to but different from the hinge regions of the γ chains. An additional tail piece follows the $C_\alpha 3$ domain and is homologous with that of the μ chain.

Homologies in the primary structure of the ε chain indicate that there are five domains (Bennich and Bahr-Lindström, 1974), but no non-domain regions related to the hinge region of the γ chain or to the tail piece of the μ chain.

IgG and IgE are found only as monomers, but IgA can be monomeric, dimeric, or tetrameric, while IgM is usually pentameric. These polymeric immunoglobulins generally have one J chain per molecule. Only immunoglobulins that have the additional tail piece exist as polymers.

Proteolytic enzymes such as pepsin, papain, and trypsin when used under carefully controlled conditions tend to cleave immunoglobulins between domains rather than within domains, although extensive degradation will occur if the digestion is prolonged. In the case of IgG, the hinge region is particularly susceptible, with Fab, $F(ab')_2$, and Fc fragments being produced (see Figure 1). IgM can be cleaved between the $C_\mu 1$ and $C_\mu 2$ domains preferentially, and between the $C_\mu2$ and $C_\mu3$ domains to give Fab, $F(ab')_2$, and $(Fc)_5$ fragments (Figure 2).

3 CRYSTALLOGRAPHIC EVIDENCE FOR DOMAINS

Several groups of X-ray crystallographers have obtained striking confirmation of the domain hypothesis. Poljak *et al.* (1972) analysed crystals of human IgG (NEW) Fab' fragment to a resolution of 0·6 nm and interpreted the results in terms of four domains. Almost simultaneously, Edmundson *et al.* (1972) analysed crystals of Bence–Jones λ chain dimer (McG) to a resolution of 0·6 nm and also interpreted their results in terms of four domains. Resolution to 0·35 nm (Schiffer *et al.*, 1973) clearly showed four globular domains and eventually a 0·23 nm model was realized (Edmundson *et al.*, 1974; Edmundson *et al.*, 1975). Higher resolution of Fab' (NEW) to 0·28 nm (Poljak *et al.*, 1973) clearly showed four globular regions (Figure 3), and further resolution provided a 0·2 nm model (Poljak *et al.*, 1974).

The four domains (V_λ, C_λ, V_H, and $C_\lambda1$) of Fab' (NEW) and the four domains (V_λ, C_λ, V_λ, C_λ) of dimer (Mcg) have a distorted tetrahedral arrangement in both cases. The angle between the pseudo two-fold axis of rotation of the V and C domains is approximately 130°. All the domains have a similar peptide chain folding, although V domains have extra folds relative to C domains formed from additional amino acid sequences (Figure 4).

Analysis of a mouse IgA (k) Fab fragment by Padlan *et al.* (1973) to a resolution of 0·45 nm showed four globular domains and the binding region for

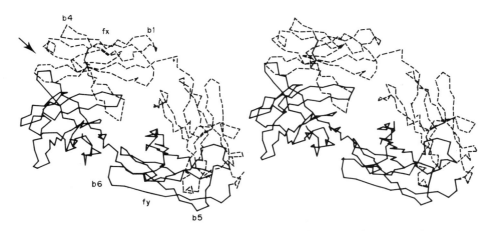

Figure 3 Stereo drawing of the 0·28 nm model of Fab' fragment of human IgG (NEW) (from Poljak *et al.*, 1973). The thin line traces the α-carbon backbone of the V_L domain (left) and the C_L domain (right). The thick line traces the α-carbon backbone of the V_H domain (left) and the $C_\gamma1$ domain (right). Note that the C_λ and $C_\gamma1$ domains have almost identical folding, and interact at their x faces. The V domains are interacting at their y faces and the antigen-binding site is indicated by an arrow. The overall dimensions of the Fab' molecule are 8 × 5 × 4 nm and those of a domain are 4 × 2·5 × 2·5 nm

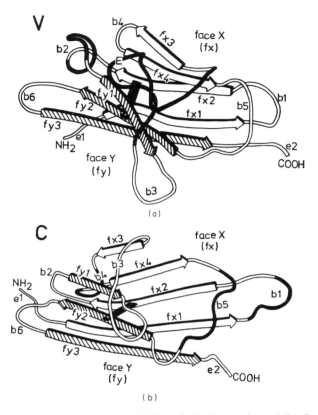

Figure 4 Peptide chain folding of (a) V domain and (b) C domain (adapted from Edmundson *et al.* 1975). The chain is folded to form seven roughly linear segments in the order fx1, fx2, fy1, fx3, fx4, fy2, and fy3. Segments fx1–4 (unshaded) and fy1–3 (shaded) form two roughly parallel faces, of anti-parallel β-pleated sheet, linked by the domain intra-chain disulphide bridge (filled rectangle). Between the β-pleated segments are other segments (b1–6) which form bends, helices, and other structure. Because of the three-dimensional tilt segments fx3, fx4, fy1, and b4 are foreshortened considerably. The V domain and the C domain differ in some of the segments b1–6 (filled in areas), in particular, V domains have an extra loop (E). The x and y faces of the V domain are more distorted than those of the C domain. The C_y1 domain is orientated to approximately the same position as the C domain shown in Figure 3.

phosphorylcholine. Subsequent resolution to 0·31 nm (Figure 5) by Segal *et al.* (1974) demonstrated that all four domains (V_κ, C_κ, V_H, $C_\alpha1$) had a similar peptide chain folding to those of Fab′ (NEW) and dimer (Mcg). Again a distorted tetrahedral arrangement of domains was observed with an angle of 135° between the pseudo two-fold axis of rotation of the V and C domains.

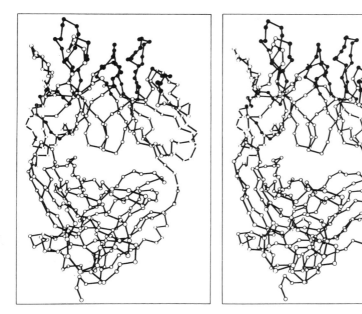

Figure 5 Stereo drawing of the 0·31 nm model of mouse (McPc 603) IgA Fab fragment (from Davies *et al.*, 1975*b*). The α-carbon backbone, –0–; hypervariable regions, –•–. The V_κ domain is top right, C_κ is bottom right, V_H is top left, and $C_\alpha1$ is bottom left. Filled circles indicate the hypervariable regions. The orientation is about 80° clockwise to that of Figure 3. Note that the C_κ and $C_\alpha1$ domains have almost identical folding which is the same as that of the C_λ and $C_\gamma1$ domains of Figure 3. The C domains are again in contact at their x faces whereas the V domains interact at their y faces

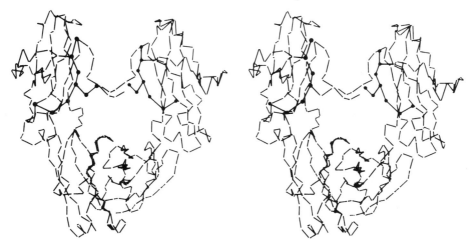

Figure 6 Stereo drawing of the α-carbon backbone of the Fc fragment from human IgG (from Deisenhofer *et al.*, 1976). The $C_\gamma2$ domains are at the top and do not interact. Approximate centres of carbohydrate units (•).

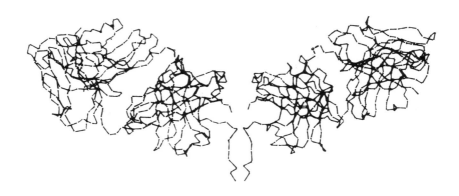

Figure 7 Tracing of the α-carbon backbone of the F(ab')₂ region from IgG1 (Kol).
From Colman *et al.*, 1976

Epp *et al.* (1974) analysed a V-region dimer to a resolution of 0·28 nm and revealed that the peptide chains fold into two globular domains. Subsequent resolution to 0·2 nm (Epp *et al.*, 1975) indicated that the two domains (V$_\kappa$, V$_\kappa$) have a similar peptide-chain folding to that of other crystallographic domains.

Analysis at 0·35 nm resolution of a human IgG Fc fragment has been reported by Deisenhofer *et al.* (1976). Four globular domains (C$_\gamma$2, C$_\gamma$3)₂ could be distinguished. These domains display a similar chain folding to those of other crystallographic models. However, C$_\gamma$2 shows some characteristic differences from other C domains (Figure 6).

X-ray crystallographic studies of whole IgG molecules generally have yielded only low resolution results which at best indicate only gross structure (Edmundson *et al.*, 1970; Sarma *et al.*, 1971). Recently, however, Colman *et al.* (1976) and Huber *et al.* (1976) have reported analysis at 0·4 nm resolution for crystals of IgG (Kol). They obtained an α carbon interpretation of the F(ab')₂ region (Figure 7), but could not resolve the Fc region which appeared to be disordered. Two points of interest to emerge were that there is no contact between the Fab arms and that the angle between the pseudo two-fold axes of rotation of V and C domains is nearly 180°, in contrast to the angle of 130° seen in Fab crystals.

4 DOMAIN STRUCTURE

Detailed comparisons of high resolution crystallographic results have been made (Davies *et al.* (1975a, b); Epp *et al* (1975); Padlan and Davies (1975); Poljak (1975a, b); Deisenhofer *et al.* (1976); Huber *et al.* (1976). In all immunoglobulin domains studied, the peptide chain is folded to form two roughly parallel, rather distorted, anti-parallel β-pleated sheets linked by the essential domain intra-chain disulphide bridge (see Figure 4). The space between the two β-pleated sheets is filled with the hydrophobic amino acid side chains, resulting in the domain interior being inaccessible to water. The two β-pleated sheets also provide the domain with two external, somewhat curved, faces (x and y in Figure 4) which are responsible for the main contacts between domains.

V Domains generally have an extra amino acid sequence, relative to C domains, which can produce various kinks or folds of different size and orientation from one V domain to another (see Davies *et al.* 1975*b*). These extra kinks or folds generally involve one of the hypervariable regions that contribute to the antigen-binding site. V_L domains have three hypervariable regions (corresponding approximately to b2, E, and b6 in Figure 4) but V_H domains have a fourth hypervariable region which is remote from the binding site (Figure 5) (see reviews by Kabat and Wu, 1971; Capra and Kehoe, 1975; Davies *et al.*, 1975*a*; Poljak, 1975*a*). The crystallographic structures of binding sites have been compared by Davies *et al.* (1975*a, b*), and Edmundson *et al.* (1975) have discussed the divergence of V and C domains.

The high resolution crystallographic data indicate that the C_λ, C_κ, $C_\gamma 1$, $C_\gamma 3$, and $C_\alpha 1$ domains have remarkably similar tertiary structures (Poljak *et al.*, 1973; Schiffer *et al.*, 1973; Segal *et al.*, 1974; Deisenhofer *et al.*, 1976) (compare Figures 3, 5, and 6) and the $C_\gamma 2$ domain has a closely related structure as shown in Figure 6 (Deisenhofer *et al.*, 1976; Huber *et al.*, 1976). Since the space between the two β-pleated sheets of a domain is filled with hydrophobic amino acid side chains, hydrophobic residues will tend to occur at alternating positions along those segments of peptide which form β-pleated sheets (fx1, 2, 3, and 4 and fy1, 2, and 3 in Figure 4). Other segments (b1, 2, 3, 4, 5, and 6) which are involved in bends, helices, and other non pleated structures do not appear to have this characteristic. Beale and Feinstein (1976) have examined the available amino acid sequences of C domains. They found that all sequences have the pattern of amino acid residues seen in the crystallographic models. This is shown in Figure 8.

It will be seen from Figure 8 (rows 1–4) that although the β-pleated and non-β-pleated segments of the V and C domains fall into approximately the same positions there are some pronounced differences. Thus in V domains, segment b1 forms a hair-pin bend, and fx1 and fx2 are displaced somewhat relative to the analogous segments of the C domains. In V domains, an extra loop occurs after b3, and fx3 is displaced relative to the analogous C domain segments. Segment b4 of V domains is considerably shorter than that of the C domains.

It will be seen from Figure 8 (columns 5–32) that in C domains the best regions of overall homology correspond to the β-pleated segments of Fab' (NEW), although it is poor in fx3 and fy3, particularly with regard to the μ and ε domains. In most of these regions, short runs of alternating hydrophobic residues tend to occur (see columns 6, 8, 10, 26, 28, 30, 32, 42, 45, 47, 66, 83, 85, 89, 91, 104, 106, 108, 119, and 124) and correspond to those with side chains pointing into the interior of the crystallographic domains.

Some of these conserved hydrophobic side chains form interesting clusters in the C_L and $C_\gamma 1$ domains of Fab' (NEW). Thus the side chains of residues in

Sample	Domain	No.	1	2	3	4	e1 (5)	6	7	8	fx1 (9)	10	11	12
Human (New) IgG₁	V_L	1					Z	S	V	L	T	Q	P	P
	V_H	2					Z	V	Q	L	P	E	S	G
	C_L	3	Q	P	K	A	A	P	S	V	T	L	F	P
	C_γ1	4	A	S	T	K	G	P	S	V	F	P	L	A
Human (Eu) IgG₁	C_γ2	5	E	L	L	G	G	P	S	V	F	L	F	P
	C_γ3	6	Q	P	—	R	E	P	Q	V	Y	T	L	P
Human (Vin) IgG₄	C_γ1	7	A	S	T	K	G	P	S	V	F	P	L	A
	C_γ2	8	E	F	L	L	G	P	S	V	F	L	F	P
	C_γ3	9	Q	P	—	R	E	P	Q	V	Y	T	L	P
Mouse (MOPC 21) IgG₁	C_γ1	10	A	K	T	T	P	P	T	V	Y	P	L	A
	C_γ2	11	E	V	—	—	—	S	S	V	F	I	F	P
	C_γ3	12	—	K	P	R	A	P	Q	V	Y	T	I	P
Mouse (MOPC 173) IgG₂ₐ	C_γ1	13	A	K	T	T	A	P	S	V	Y	P	L	A
	C_γ2	14	N	L	L	G	G	P	S	V	F	I	F	P
	C_γ3	15	—	S	V	R	A	P	Q	V	Y	V	L	P
Guinea pig IgG₂	C_γ1	16	A	S	T	T	A	P	S	V	F	P	L	A
	C_γ2	17	E	N	L	G	G	P	S	V	F	I	F	P
	C_γ3	18	—	A	P)	R	M	P	D	V	Y	T	L	P
Rabbit IgG	C_γ1	19	S	G	T	K	A	P	S	V	F	P	L	A
	C_γ2	20	E	L	L	G	G	P	S	V	F	I	F	K
	C_γ3	21	E	P	L	—	E	P	K	V	Y	T	M	G
Human (Gal) IgM	C_μ1	22	G	S	A	S	A	P	T	L	F	P	L	V
	C_μ2	23	Z	L	P	P	K	V	S	V	F	V	P	P
	C_μ3	24	D	Z	B	T	A	I	R	V	F	A	I	P
	C_μ4	25	V	A	L	H	R	P	D	V		L	L	P
Human (ND) IgE	C_ε1	26	G	S	T	T	G	P	T	V	F)	P	L	T
	C_ε2	27	R	B	F	T	P	P	T	V	K	I	L	Z
	C_ε3	28	A	D	S	D	P	R	G	V	S	A	Y	L
	C_ε4	29	G	P	R	A	A	P	E	V	Y	A	F	A
Human IgA₁	C_α1	30	A	S	P	T	S	P	K	V	F	P	L	S
	C_α2	31	P	S	C	C	H	P	R	L	S	L	H	R
	C_α3	32	—	N	T	F	H	P	E	V	R	L	L	P
Human (Mcg)	C_L	33	Q	P	K	A	N	P	T	V	T	L	F	P
	V_L	34					Z	S	A	L	T	Q	P	P
β-microglob'		35	—	I	Q	R	T	P	K	I	Q	V	Y	S

Single-letter

A	alanine (n)	G	glycine (n)
B	aspartic-acid or asparagine	H	histidine
		I	isoleucine (h)
C	cysteine	K	lysine
D	aspartic acid	L	leucine (h)
E	glutamic acid	M	methionine(h)
F	phenylalanine (h)	N	asparagine

Figure 8 Alignment of amino acid sequences in terms of crystallographic models. In rows 1–4 the amino acid sequences of the four domains of Fab' (NEW) are aligned by the method of Poljak et al. (1974) with residues occupying equivalent positions in the 0·2 nm model placed in the same column. Hydrogen-bonded residues are indicated by cancelled

```
                              b1                               fx2
S   V   S   G   A   P   —   —   —   —   G   Q   R   V   T   I   S   C   T
P   E   L   V   S   P   —   —   —   —   G   Z   T   L   S   L   T   C   T
P   S   S   E   E   L   Q   —   —   —   A   N   K   A   T   L   V   C   L
P   S   S   K   S   T   S   —   —   —   G   G   T   A   A   L   G   C   L
▼
                              20                              30
P   K   P   K   D   T   —   L   M   I   S   R   T   P   E   V   T   C   V
P   S   R   E   E   —   —   —   M   T   K   N   Q   V   S   L   T   C   L

P   C   S   R   T   S   —   —   —   E   S   T   A   A   L   G   C   L
P   K   P   K   D   T   —   L   M   I   S   R   T   P   E   V   T   C   V
P   S   Q   E   E   —   —   —   M   T   K   N   Q   V   S   L   T   C   L

P   G   S   N   A   A   S   —   —   —   Q   S   M   V   T   L   G   C   L
P   K   P   K   D   T   —   L   L   I   T   V   T   P   K   V   T   C   V
P   P   K   E   Q   —   —   —   M   A   K   D   K   V   S   L   T   C   M

P   V   C   G   D   T   T   —   —   —   G   S   S   V   T   L   G   C   L
V   K   I   K   N   P   —   L   M   I   S   L   S   P   I   V   T   C   V
P   P   Z   S   —   —   —   —   M   T   K   K   E   V   T   L   T   C   M

A   S   C   V   D   T   S   —   —   —   G   S   M   M   T   L   G   C   L
P   K   P   K   D   T   —   L   M   I   S   L   T   P   R   V   T   C   V
P   S   R   D   E   —   —   —   L   S   K   S   K   V   S   V   T   C   L

P   C   C   G   D   T   P   —   —   —   S   S   T   V   T   L   G   C   L
P   P   P   K   D   T   —   L   M   I   S   R   T   P   E   V   T   C   V
P   P   R   E   Q   —   —   —   L   S   S   R   S   V   S   L   T   C   M

S   C   E   N   S   B   P   —   —   —   S   S   T   V   A   V   G   C   L
R   D   G   F   F   G   N   —   —   —   P   R   K   S   K   L   I   C   Q
P   S   F   A   S   —   —   I   F   L   T   K   S   T   K   L   T   C   L
P   A   R   E   Q   —   —   L   N   L   R   E   S   A   T   I   T   C   L

R   C   C   K   B   I   P   —   S   N   A   T   S   V   T   L   G   C   L
S   S   C   B   G   L   —   —   G   H   F   P   P   T   I   Z   L   C   L
S   R   P   S   P   F   D   L   F   I   R   K   S   P   T   I   T   C   L
T   P   E   W   P   G   S   —   —   —   R   D   K   R   T   L   A   C   L

L   C   S   T   Z   P   —   —   —   —   B   G   B   V   V   I   A   C   L
P   A   L   Q   D   —   —   L   L   L   G   S   E   A   N   L   T   C   T
P   P   S   Q   Q   —   —   L   A   L   N   Q   L   V   T   L   T   C   L
▲                                           ▲       ▲       ▲
P   S   S   E   E   L   Q   —   —   —   A   N   K   A   T   L   V   C   L
S   A   S   G   S   L   —   —   —   —   G   Q   S   V   T   I   S   C   T
R   H   P   A   E   N   —   —   —   —   G   K   S   N   F   L   N   C   Y
```

amino acid code:

P	proline (h)	W	tryptophan
Q	glutamine	Y	tyrosine
R	arginine	Z	glutamic acid
S	serine		or glutamine
T	threonine		
V	valine (h)	(n)	non-polar
		(h)	hydrophobic

letters. Segments participating in pleated sheets are underlined and labelled fx1–4 and fy1–3, in accordance with Figure 4. Segments forming bends, helices, or other structure are labelled b1–6. Residues of other structure at the ends of the domain are e1 and e2. $C_\gamma 1$. Residues whose side chains point to the interior of the domain have a filled triangle

Column markers: **b2** (above column 9), **fy1** (above column 13); **40** refers to columns between rows 4 and 5.

	1	2	3	4	5	6	7	8	9	10	11	12	13	14	15
Human (New) IgG₁	G	S	S	S	N	I	—	—	G	A	G	N	H	V	K
	G	S	T	V	S	T	—	—	F	A	V	—	Y	I	V
	I	S	D	F	Y	P	—	—	G	A	V	—	T	V	A
	V	K	D	Y	F	P	—	—	E	P	V	—	T	V	S
Human (Eu) IgG₁	V	V	D	V	S	H	E	D	P	Q	V	—	K	F	N
	V	K	G	F	Y	P	—	—	S	D	I	—	A	V	E
Human (Vin) IgG₄	V	K	.	.	.	.	.	.	.	.	.	.	.	.	.
	V	V	D	V	S	Q	E	D	P	Z	(V	—	Z	F)	N
	V	K	G	F	Y	P	—	—	S	D	I	—	A	V	E
Mouse (MOPC 21) IgG₁	V	K	G	Y	F	P	—	—	E	P	V	—	T	V	T
	V	V	D	I	S	K	D	D	P	E	V	—	Q	F	S
	I	T	D	F	F	P	—	—	E	D	I	—	T	V	E
Mouse (MOPC 173) IgG₂ₐ	V	K	G	Y	F	P	—	—	E	P	V	—	T	L	S
	V	V	D	V	S	E	D	D	P	D	V	—	Q	I	S
	V	T	N	F	M	P	—	—	E	D	I	—	Y	V	E
Guinea pig IgG₂	V	K	G	Y	F	P	—	—	E	P	V	—	T	V	K
	V	V	D	V	S	Q	D	E	P	E	V	—	Q	F	T
	L	I	N	F	F	P	—	—	A	D	I	—	H	V	E
Rabbit IgG	V	K	G	Y	L	P	—	—	E	P	V	—	T	V	T
	V	V	D	V	S	Z	B	(D	P	Z	V	—	Z)	F	T
	I	D	G	F	Y	P	—	—	S	D	I	—	S	V	G
Human (Gal) IgM	A	Z	D	F	L	P	—	—	D	S	I	—	T	F	S
	A	T	G	F	S	P	—	—	R	Q	I	—	Q	V	S
	V	T	D	L	T	Y	—	—	D	S	V	—	T	I	S
	V	T	G	F	S	P	—	—	A	D	V	—	F	V	Q
Human (ND) IgE	A	T	G	Y	F	P	—	—	E	P	V	—	M	V	T
	V	S	G	Y	T	P	—	—	G	T	I	—	𝒩	I	T
	V	V	B	L	A	P	S	K	G	T	V	—	𝒩	L	T
	I	Q	N	F	M	P	—	—	E	D	I	—	S	V	Q
Human IgA₁	V	Q	G	F	F	P	—	Q	Q	P	L	—	S	V	T
	L	T	G	L	R	D	—	A	S	G	V	—	T	F	T
	A	R	G	F	S	P	—	—	K	D	V	—	L	V	R
Human (Mcg)	I	S	D	F	Y	P	—	—	G	A	V	—	T	V	A
	G	T	S	S	D	V	—	—	G	G	Y	N	Y	V	S
β-microglob'	V	S	G	F	H	P	—	—	S	D	I	—	E	V	D

Single-letter

A	alanine (n)	G	glycine (n)
B	aspartic-acid or asparagine	H	histidine
C	cysteine	I	isoleucine (h)
D	aspartic acid	K	lysine
E	glutamic acid	L	leucine (h)
F	phenylalanine (h)	M	methionine (h)
		N	asparagine

underneath. Rows 5–32, available amino acid sequences of C_H domains aligned by homology, which has been maximized by leaving gaps (–). The numbering between rows 4 and 5 refers to columns not to residues. C, Cysteine residues; 𝒩, sites for complex N-linked oligosaccharide; S, sites for O-linked carbohydrate. Columns which tend to conserve

The sequence alignment table (with β-strand label b3, the "extra loop" region, and residue numbering 50 and 60):

		50			b3				extra loop				60				
W	Y	Q	Q	L	P	G	T										
W	V	R	Q	P	P	G	R						P	L	R	S	R
W	K	—	—	A	D	S	S	—	—	—	—	—	P	V	K	A	—
W	N	—	—	—	S	G	—	—	—	—	—	—	A	L	T	S	—

▼

W	Y	—	—	V	D	G	—	—	—	—	—	—	V	Q	V	H	
W	E	—	—	S	N	D	—	—	—	—	—	—	G	E	P	E	—
.	.	.	.	.	.	.	.	.	.								.
W	Y	—	—	V	D	G	—	—	—	—	—	—	V	E	V	H	—
W	Z	—	—	S	(B	B	—	—	—	—	—	—	G	Z	P	Z	—
W	N	—	—	—	S	G	—	—	—	—	—	—	S	L	S	S	—
W	F	—	—	V	D	N	—	—	—	—	—	—	V	E	V	H	—
W	E	—	—	S	N	G	—	—	—	—	—	—	Q	A	P	E	—
W	T	—	—	—	L	G	—	—	—	—	—	—	B	S	S	S	—
W	F	—	—	V	D	N	—	—	—	—	—	—	V	E	V	H	—
W	T	—	—	N	N	G	—	—	—	—	—	—	K	T	E	L	—
W	N	—	—	—	S	G	—	—	—	—	—	—	A	L	T	S	—
W	F	—	—	V	D	N	—	—	—	—	—	—	K	P	V	G	—
W	A	—	—	S	N	R	—	—	—	V	P	V	S	E	K	—	
W	N	—	—	—	S	G	—	—	—	—	—	—	T	L	T	D	—
W	Y	—	—	I	B	B	—	—	—	—	—	—	Z	Q	V	R	—
W	E	—	—	K	D	G	—	—	—	—	—	—	K	A	E	D	—
W	K	—	—	Y	K	*N*	—	—	—	—	—	N	S	D	I	S	—
W	L	—	—	R	E	G	—	—	—	—	—	K	Q	V	G	S	—
W	T	—	—	R	Q	D	—	—	—	—	—	—	G	E	—	—	—
W	Q	—	—	M	Q	R	—	—	—	—	G	Q	P	L	S	P	E
W	B	—	—	—	T	G	—	—	—	—	—	—	S	L	*N*	—	—
W	L	—	—	Z	B	G	—	—	—	—	—	—	Z	V	M	—	—
W	S	—	—	R	A	S	—	—	—	—	—	—	G	K	—	—	—
W	L	—	—	H	N	E	—	—	—	—	—	—	V	Q	L	P	—
W	S	—	—	—	Z	S	—	—	—	—	—	—	G	Z	G	V	—
W	T	—	—	—	P	S	—	—	—	—	—	—	S	G	K	S	—
W	L	—	—	Q	G	S	—	—	—	—	—	Q	E	L	P	R	E

▲   ▲

W	K	—	—	A	D	G	S						P	V	K	—	—
W	Y	Q	Q	H	A	G	K						—	—	—	—	R
L	L	—	—	K	D	G	—	—	—	—	—	—	E	R	I	—	—

amino acid code:

P	proline (h)	W	tryptophan
Q	glutamine	Y	tyrosine
R	arginine	Z	glutamic acid
S	serine		or glutamine
T	threonine		
V	valine (h)	(n)	non-polar
		(h)	hydrophobic

hydrophobic residues at alternating positions are shown by sans serif letters. A column in which serine residues are largely conserved is similarly shown. Rows 33 and 34, the domains of Bence–Jones dimer (Mcg) have been aligned using the results of Edmundson *et al.* (1975). Residues having extended structure, mainly involved in β-pleated sheets are

			fx3											b4	
Human (New)	~~F~~	~~S~~	~~V~~	~~S~~	K	~~S~~	G	—	—	—	—	—	—	—	—
IgG$_1$	V	~~T~~	M	~~L~~	V	N	T	—	S	—	—	—	—	—	—
	—	~~G~~	V	~~E~~	T	~~T~~	T	P	~~S~~	K	~~Q~~	—	—	S	N
	—	~~G~~	V	~~H~~	T	~~F~~	P	A	~~V~~	L	~~Q~~	—	—	S	S
			▼		▼										
							70								
Human (Eu)	—	N	**A**	K	T	K	P	R	E	Q	Q	—	—	Y	$\mathcal{N}$
IgG$_1$	—	N	**Y**	K	T	T	P	P	V	L	D	—	—	S	D
Human (Vin)	.	.	.	.	.	.	.	.	.	.	.	.	.	.	.
IgG$_4$	—	N	**A**	K	T	K	P	R	E	E	Q	—	—	F	$\mathcal{N}$
	—	B	**Y)**	K	T	T	P	P	V	L	D	—	—	S	D
Mouse (MOPC	—	G	**V**	H	T	F	P	A	V	L	Q	—	—	S	D
21) IgG$_1$	—	T	**A**	Q	T	Q	P	R	E	E	Q	—	—	F	$\mathcal{N}$
	—	N	**Y**	K	N	T	Q	P	I	M	D	—	—	T	D
Mouse (MOPC	—	G	**V**	H	T	F	P	A	V	L	Q	—	—	S	D
173) IgG$_{2a}$	—	Q	**A**	Q	T	T	H	T	R	Q	N	—	—	Y	$\mathcal{N}$
	—	N	**Y**	K	N	T	Q	P	V	L	D	—	—	S	D
Guinea pig	—	G	**V**	H	T	F	P	A	V	L	Q	—	—	S	G
IgG$_2$	—	N	A	E	T	K	P	R	V	E	Q	—	—	Y	$\mathcal{N}$
	—	E	**Y**	K	N	T	P	P	I	E	D	—	—	A	D
Rabbit IgG	—	G	**V**	R	T	F	P	S	V	R	Q	—	—	S	S
	—	T	**A**	R	P	P	L	R	E	Q	Q	—	—	F	$\mathcal{N}$
	—	D	Y	K	T	T	P	A	V	L	D	—	—	S	D
Human (Gal)	—	S	**T**	R	G	F	P	S	V	L	R	—	—	G	G
IgM	—	G	**V**	T	T	N	E	V	Z	A	Z	A	K	E	S
	—	A	**V**	K	T	H	T	$\mathcal{N}$	I	S	Z	S	H	P	$\mathcal{N}$
	—	K	**Y**	V	T	S	A	P	M	P	E	P	Q	A	P
Human (ND)	—	G	**T**	T	L	P	A	T	T	L	T	—	—	L	S
IgE	—	D	**V**	D	L	S	T	A	S	T	E	—	—	S	E
	—	P	**V**	B	H	S	T	R	K	E	E	K	Q	R	$\mathcal{N}$
	—	D	**A**	R	H	S	T	T	Q	P	R	K	T	K	G
Human IgA$_1$	—	T	**A**	R	B	F	P	P	S	Z	B	—	—	A	S
	—	A	**V**	Q	G	P	P	B	R	D	L	—	—	**C**	G
	—	K	**Y**	L	T	W	A	S	R	Q	Q	P	S	Q	G
			▲		▲			▲							
Human (Mcg)	A	G	V	E	T	T	K	P	S	K	Q	—	—	S	N
	F	S	G	S	K	S	G	—	—	—	—	—	—	—	—
β-microglob	E	K	V	E	H	S	D	L	S	F	—	—	—	S	K

Single-letter

A	alanine (n)	G	glycine (n)
B	aspartic-acid or asparagine	H	histidine
		I	isoleucine (h)
C	cysteine	K	lysine
D	aspartic acid	L	leucine (h)
E	glutamic acid	M	methionine (h)
F	phenylalanine (h)	N	asparagine

underlined. Residue whose side chains point to the interior of the C_L domain are marked at the top by a filled triangle. hr, hinge region. tp, extra-domain tail piece. Amino acid sequences were obtained from: human IgG1 (NEW)—Poljak *et al.* (1974); human IgG1 (Eu), human IgG4 (Vin), and rabbit IgG—Dayhoff (1972), Croft (1974); mouse IgG1—

						fx4												b5
—	—	—	—	—	—	S	S	A	T	L	A	I	T	G	L	Q	—	—
—	—	—	—	—	K	N	Q	F	S	L	R	L	S	S	V	T	—	—
N	—	—	K	Y	A	A	S	S	Y	L	S	L	T	P	E	Q	—	—
G	—	—	L	Y	S	L	S	S	V	V	T	V	P	S	S	—	—	—
						▼		▼		▼		▼						

			80										90					
S	—	—	T	Y	R	V	V	S	V	L	T	V	L	H	Q	N	—	—
G	—	—	S	F	F	L	Y	S	K	L	T	V	D	K	S	R	—	—
.		.		.										.		.		.
S	—	—	T	Y	R	V	(V	S	V	L	T	V	L	H	Z	B	—	—
G	—	—	S	F	F	L	Y	S	R	L	T	V	D	K	S	R	—	—
—	—	—	L	Y	T	L	S	S	S	V	S	V	P	T	S	P	—	—
S	—	—	T	F	R	V	V	S	A	L	P	I	M	H	Q	D	—	—
G	—	—	S	Y	F	V	Y	S	K	L	N	V	Q	K	S	N	—	—
—	—	—	L	Y	S	S	S	V	T	V	T	V	T	S	S	S	T	—
S	—	—	T	L	R	V	V	S	A	L	P	I	Q	H	Q	N	—	—
G	—	—	S	Y	F	M	Y	S	K	L	R	V	E	K	K	N	—	—
—	—	—	L	Y	S	L	T	S	M	V	T	V	P	S	S	Q	—	—
T	—	—	T	F	R	V	E	S	V	L	P	I	Q	H	Q	D	—	—
G	—	—	S	Y	F	L	Y	S	K	L	T	V	D	K	S	A	—	—
G	—	—	L	Y	S	V	P	S	T	V	S	V	S	Z	P	—	—	—
S	—	—	T	I	R	V	V	S	T	L	P	I	A	H	E	D	—	—
G	—	—	S	W	F	L	Y	S	K	L	S	V	P	T	S	E	—	—
—	—	—	K	Y	A	A	T	S	Q	V	L	L	P	S	K	D	V	M
G	P	T	T	Y	K	V	T	S	T	L	T	I	K	E	S	B	—	—
A	—	—	T	F	S	A	V	G	E	A	S	I	C	E	B	B	—	—
G	—	—	R	Y	F	A	H	S	I	L	T	V	S	E	E	E	—	—
G	—	—	H	Y	A	T	I	S	L	L	T	V	S	G	A	—	—	—
G	E	—	L	A	S	T	E	S	E	L	T	L	S	Q	K	H	—	—
G	—	—	T	L	T	V	T	S	T	L	P	V	G	T	R	B	—	—
S	—	—	G	F	F	V	S	R	L	E	V	T	R	A	E	—	—	—
G	B	—	L	Y	T	T	S	S	Q	L	T	L	P	A	T	Z	C	—
C	—	—	—	Y	S	V	S	S	V	L	P	G	C	A	Q	P	—	—
T	E	—	T	F	A	V	T	S	I	L	R	V	A	A	E	D	—	—
						▲		▲		▲		▲						
N	—	—	K	Y	A	A	S	S	Y	L	S	L	T	P	E	Q	—	—
—	—	—	—	—	N	T	A	S	L	T	V	S	G	L	Q	—	—	—
N	W	—	S	F	Y	L	L	Y	S	Y	T	E	F	T	P	T	—	—

amino acid code:

P	proline (h)	W	tryptophan
Q	glutamine	Y	tyrosine
R	arginine	Z	glutamic acid
S	serine		or glutamine
T	threonine		
V	valine (h)	(n)	non-polar
		(h)	hydrophobic

Milstein *et al.* (1974), Adetugbo *et al.* (1975); mouse IgG2a—Bourgois *et al.* (1974), Rocca-Serra *et al.* (1975); guinea-pig IgG2—Tracy and Cebra (1974), Trischmann and Cebra (1974); human IgM (Gal)—Watanabe *et al.* (1973); human IgE (ND)—Bennich and Bahr-Lindström (1974); human IgA1—Kratzin *et al.* (1976); Bence–Jones dimer (Mcg)—Edmundson *et al.* (1975); β-microglobulin—Cunningham (1974)

								fy2							b6
Human (New) IgG₁	~~A~~	E	~~D~~	~~E~~	~~A~~	~~D~~	~~Y~~	~~Y~~	~~C~~	Q	~~S~~	~~Y~~	~~D~~	R	S
	~~A~~	A	~~D~~	~~T~~	~~A~~	~~V~~	~~Y~~	~~Y~~	~~C~~	A	R	~~B~~	~~L~~	I	A
	W	K	S	H	~~K~~	S	~~Y~~	~~S~~	~~C~~	Q	~~V~~	~~T~~	~~H~~	—	—
	—	L	G	T	Q	T	~~Y~~	~~I~~	~~C~~	~~N~~	~~V~~	~~N~~	~~H~~	K	P
							▼		▼		▼		▼		

			100										110		
Human (Eu) IgG₁	W	L	D	G	K	E	Y	K	C	K	V	S	N	K	A
	W	Q	Q	G	N	V	F	S	C	S	V	M	H	E	A
Human (Vin) IgG₄	.	.	.	.	.	T	Y	T	C	N	V	D	H	K	P
	W	L	B	G)	K	E	Y	K	C	K	V	S	N	K	G
	(W	Z	Z	G	B	V	F	S	C	S	V	M	(H	Z	A
Mouse (MOPC 21) IgG₁	—	—	—	—	E	T	V	T	C	N	V	A	H	A	P
	W	L	N	G	K	E	F	K	C	R	V	N	S	A	A
	W	Q	A	G	N	T	F	T	C	S	V	L	H	E	G
Mouse (MOPC 173) IgG₂ₐ	W	P	S	Q	S	I	T	N	C	N	V	A	H	P	A
	W	M	S	G	K	E	F	K	C	K	V	N	N	K	D
	W	V	E	R	N	S	F	S	C	S	V	V	H	Q	G
Guinea pig IgG₂	—	—	—	—	—	K	A	T	C	N	V	A	H	P	A
	W	L	R	G	K	E	F	K	C	K	V	Y	N	K	A
	W	D	Q	G	T	V	Y	T	C	S	V	M	H	E	A
Rabbit IgG	—	—	—	—	—	(P	S)	T	C	B	V	A	H	A	(T
	W	L	R	G	K	E	F	K	C	K	V	H	D	K	A
	W	Q	R	G	D	V	F	T	C	S	V	M	H	E	A
Human (Gal) IgM	Q	G	T	N	E	H	V	V	C	K	V	Z	H	P	B
	W	L	S	Q	S	M	F	T	C	R	V	D	H	R	G
	W	N	S	G	E	R	F	T	C	T	V	T	H	T	D
	W	N	T	G	E	T	Y	T	C	V	V	A	H	E	A
Human (ND) IgE	W	A	K	—	Q	M	F	T	C	R	V	A	H	—	—
	W	L	S	D	R	T	Y	Z	C	E	V	T	Y	—	—
	W	I	E	G	E	T	Y	Z	C	R	V	T	H	P	H
	W	Q	E	K	D	E	F	I	C	R	A	V	H	E	A
Human IgA₁	—	L	A	G	K	S	V	T	C	H	V	K	H	—	—
	W	N	H	G	K	T	F	T	C	T	A	A	Y	P	E
	W	K	K	G	D	T	F	S	C	M	V	G	H	E	A
	▲					▲		▲		▲		▲			
Human (Mcg)	W	K	S	H	R	S	Y	S	C	Q	V	T	H	—	—
	A	E	D	E	A	D	Y	Y	C	S	S	Y	E	G	S
β-microglob'	—	E	K	—	D	E	Y	A	C	R	V	N	H	—	—

Single-letter

A	alanine (n)	G	glycine (n)
B	aspartic-acid or asparagine	H	histidine
		I	isoleucine (h)
C	cysteine	K	lysine
D	aspartic acid	L	leucine (h)
E	glutamic acid	M	methionine (h)
F	phenylalanine (h)	N	asparagine

						fy3									e2				
—	—	—	L	R	—	V	F	G	G	G	T	K	L	T	V	L	R	1	V_L
G	—	—	C	I	B	V	W	G	Q	G	S	L	V	T	V	S	S	2	V_H
E	G	—	S	T	—	V	B	K	T	—	V	A	P	T	E	C	S	3	C_L
S	N	—	T	K	—	V	D	K	R	—	V	E	P	K	S	C	hr	4	$C_\gamma 1$

▼ (under col 4) ▼ (under col 11)   **120**

L	P	—	A	P	—	I	E	K	T	—	I	S	K	A	K	G		5	$C_\gamma 2$
L	H	N	H	Y	—	T	Q	K	S	—	L	S	L	S	P	G		6	$C_\gamma 3$
S	N	—	T	K	—	V	D	K	R	—	V	E	S	K	Y	G	hr	7	$C_\gamma 1$
L	P	—	S	S	—	I	E	K	T	—	I	S	K	A	K	G		8	$C_\gamma 2$
L	H	B	H	Y)	—	T	Q	K	S	—	L	S	L	S	L	G		9	$C_\gamma 3$
S	S	—	T	K	—	V	D	K	K	—	I	V	P	R	D	C	hr	10	$C_\gamma 1$
F	P	—	A	P	—	I	E	K	T	—	I	S	K	T	K	G		11	$C_\gamma 2$
L	H	N	H	H	—	T	E	K	S	—	L	S	H	S	P	G		12	$C_\gamma 3$
S	S	—	T	K	—	V	D	K	K	—	I	E	P	R	G	P	hr	13	$C_\gamma 1$
L	P	—	A	P	—	I	E	R	T	—	I	S	K	P	K	G		14	$C_\gamma 2$
L	H	N	H	V	—	S	T	K	S	—	F	S	R	T	P	G		15	$C_\gamma 3$
S	S	—	T	K	—	V	D	K	T	—	V	E	P	I	R	T	hr	16	$C_\gamma 1$
L	P	—	A	P	—	I	E	K	T	—	I	S	K	T	K	G		17	$C_\gamma 2$
L	H	N	H	V	—	T	Q	K	A	—	I	S	R	S	P	G		18	$C_\gamma 3$
B)	—	—	T	K	—	V	D	K	T	—	V	A	P	S	T	C	hr	19	$C_\gamma 1$
L	P	—	A	P	—	I	E	K	T	—	I	S	K	A	R	G		20	$C_\gamma 2$
L	H	N	H	Y	—	T	Q	K	S	—	I	S	R	S	P	G		21	$C_\gamma 3$
G	B	—	K	E	—	K	D	V	P	—	L	P	V	I	A	—		22	$C_\mu 1$
—	—	—	L	T	—	F	Q	Q	*N*	—	A	S	S	M	C	V	P	23	$C_\mu 2$
L	P	—	S	P	—	L	K	Q	T	—	I	S	R	P	K	G		24	$C_\mu 3$
L	P	N	R	V	—	T	E	R	T	—	V	D	K	S	T	G	tp	25	$C_\mu 4$
T	P	—	S	S	—	T	B	*N*	V	—	K	T	F	S	V	C	S	26	$C_\varepsilon 1$
Z	G	←	H	T	—	F	Z	B	S	—	T	K	K	C	—	—		27	$C_\varepsilon 2$
L	P	—	R	A	—	L	M	R	S	—	T	T	K	T	S	—		28	$C_\varepsilon 3$
A	S	P	S	Q	—	T	V	Q	R	A	V	S	V	N	P	G	K	29	$C_\varepsilon 4$
Y	T	—	B	P	—	S	Z	B	V	—	T	V	P	C	—	—	hr	30	$C_z 1$
—	—	—	S	K	—	T	P	L	T	A	T	L	S	K	S	G		31	$C_z 2$
L	P	L	A	F	—	T	Q	K	T	—	I	D	R	L	A	G	tp	32	$C_z 3$

▲ (under col 4) ▲ (under col 11)

E	G	—	S	T	—	V	E	K	—	T	V	A	P	T	E	C	S	33	C_L
D	—	—	N	F	—	V	F	G	T	G	T	K	V	T	V	L	G	34	V_L
V	T	—	L	S	—	Q	P	K	I	—	V	K	W	D	R	D	M	35	

amino acid code:

P	proline (h)	W	tryptophan
Q	glutamine	Y	tyrosine
R	arginine	Z	glutamic acid
S	serine		or glutamine
T	threonine		
V	valine (h)	(n)	non-polar
		(h)	hydrophobic

columns 8, 32, 108, and 119 in Figure 8 are in close proximity in the three-dimensional model and involve segments fx1, fx2, fy2, and fy3. Similarly, the side chains of residues in columns 28, 66, and 89 are near to each other and involve segments fx2, fx3, and fx4. The tendency to form such hydrophobic clusters probably influences the pattern of folding of the domains. Regions of the C-domain sequences which correspond to non-β-pleated segments of the crystallographic models have very little overall homology.

Examination of V-domain sequences (Dayhoff, 1972) shows that some of the conserved hydrophobic sites found in C domains also occur in V domains (see columns 6, 8, 26, 28, 30, 45, 47, 89, 91, 104, and 106), but others do not. On the other hand, V domains tend to conserve hydrophobic residues at some positions where C domains do not (columns 14, 16, 64, 87, 94, 126, and 128). Different hydrophobic clusters are produced therefore. For example, in V_L (NEW) the side chains of residues in columns 14, 26, 91, 94, 126, and 128 are in close proximity. Another cluster involves side chains from residues in columns 28, 47, 66, 89, and 104, and two sites in the loop which C domains do not have. Such differences in hydrophobic clustering probably influence the differences in chain-folding between V and C domains.

From this discussion, it appears highly probable that the C domains shown in rows 5–32 of Figure 8 would have the same basic immunoglobulin fold as that seen in high-resolution crystallographic models. Also, it is likely that these C domains would have more of the characteristics of the crystallographic C domains than of the V domains.

Some C domains appear to have conserved certain sequence features, thus suggesting the possibility of specialized folding in localized regions of the domain. From Figure 8 it will be seen that $C_\gamma 2$, $C_\mu 3$, and $C_\varepsilon 3$ have three consecutive hydrophobic residues in segment b1 (columns 20–22). Furthermore, most C domains have a noticeably conserved triplet of residues in columns 35–37 consisting of an aromatic, a hydrophobic and proline residue. $C_\gamma 2$, $C_\mu 3$, and $C_\alpha 2$ clearly lack this feature of segment b2. $C_\gamma 2$, $C_\alpha 2$ and $C_\mu 2$ domains do not have a histidine residue (H) in column 110 as do other C domains.

Regions where homology is very poor, such as columns 58–81 in Figure 8 may have undergone specialized folding, particularly in C_μ and C_ε domains. Even when homology is good there can be some unexpected differences in peptide chain folding. Thus, Deisenhofer *et al.* (1976) and Huber *et al.* (1976) have reported that, although most of the $C_\gamma 2$ domain has a remarkably similar folding to that of $C_\gamma 3$ and $C_\gamma 1$, there are significant variations in two of the bends and two of the β-pleated segments. In Figures 4 and 8, these differences would involve b3, fx3, b4, and fx4. Although homology between $C_\gamma 2$ and $C_\gamma 3$ is very good from columns 65 to 70 of Figure 8, the peptide-chain folding is significantly different. In $C_\gamma 3$, these residues form part of the β-pleated segment fx3 as in $C_\gamma 1$ and C_L, whereas in $C_\gamma 2$, they form an extension to b3 to give an extra kink somewhat reminiscent of V domains. Segment fx3 consequently is shortened and displaced in $C_\gamma 2$ relative to the analogous segment in $C_\gamma 3$, $C_\gamma 1$, and C_L. Accompanying displacements of b4 and fx4 also occur. Huber *et al.* (1976) have pointed out that the differences result in these segments showing some resemblance to V-domain folding.

5 DISULPHIDE BRIDGES

Each domain has an intra-domain disulphide bridge. It lies in the hydrophobic space between the domain faces and is therefore inaccessible to thiol-reducing agents in aqueous solution. The light-chain cysteine residue which participates in the light–heavy disulphide bridge is situated at the C-terminal end of the C_L domain (segment e2 of Figure 4; rows 3, 33 of Figure 8). In human and mouse IgG1, the heavy-chain cysteine residue completing this light–heavy disulphide bridge lies at the C-terminal end of the $C_\gamma 1$ domain (segment e2 of Figure 4; rows 4 and 10 of Figure 8). In all other immunoglobulins shown in Figure 8, the light–heavy bridge is completed by a cysteine residue lying in segment b1 of the $C_\gamma 1$, $C_\mu 1$, $C_\varepsilon 1$, or $C_\alpha 1$ domains (columns 14 or 15, Figure 8). Examination of the crystallographic models shows that e2 and b1 are in close spatial proximity (Figure 9). Rabbit IgG and human IgE have an additional intra-chain disulphide bridge. This bond is accessible to thiol reagents in aqueous solution. In both cases, the cysteine residues which form this bridge lie in segments b1 and e2 (rows 19 and 26, columns 14 or 15 and 129; Figure 8) which are in close proximity (Figure 9). IgA probably has additional intra-chain disulphide bridges, which are accessible to reducing agents, linking b5 and e2 in the $C_\alpha 1$ domain (row 30, columns 14 and 127, Figure 8; Figure 9) and linking b4 to e1 in the $C_\alpha 2$ domain (row 31, columns 4 and 27, Figure 8; Figure 9).

The inter-heavy chain disulphide bridges of IgG lie in the non-domain hinge region (see Figure 10). IgM has no such region but has a symmetrical bridge at the C-terminal end of the $C_\mu 2$ domain in segment e2 (row 23, column 128, Figure 8; Figure 10). There is also a μ bridge between μ chains at b5 in the $C_\mu 3$ domain of human IgM, and this was thought to act as the only inter-subunit bridge (Beale and Feinstein, 1969, 1970; Miekka and Deutsch, 1970). In contrast the inter-μ-chain bridge in the extra-domain tail piece (Figure 10) was thought to be intra-subunit; however more recent evidence (Feinstein et al., 1976) has shown that this extra-domain bridge is also inter-subunit, as in Figure 2. The $C_\mu 3$ bridge has not been detected in mouse IgM (Milstein et al., 1975). IgE also has no hinge region analogous to that of IgG. There are, however, two inter-ε chain bridges in segments b1 and b2 of the $C_\varepsilon 2$ domain (row 27, columns 15 and 127, Figure 8; Figure 10). IgA possibly has inter-heavy chain bridges at e1 or b4 of the $C_\alpha 2$ domains (row 31, Figure 8; Figure 9). Cysteine residues in b5 of the $C_\alpha 2$ domain and in the non-domain tail piece also probably from inter-α-chain bridges one of which may be involved in polymerization (row 31, Figure 8; Figure 9).

6 OLIGOSACCHARIDE SITES

All immunoglobulin heavy chains contain N-linked oligosaccharide and there appears to be an homologous site in segment b4 of $C_\gamma 2$, $C_\mu 3$, and $C_\varepsilon 3$ domains,

282

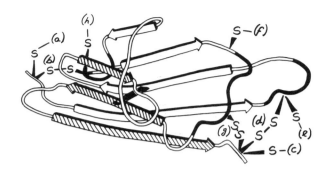

Figure 9 Location of disulphide bridges on
the three-dimensional model of the C
domain (adapted from Edmundson *et al.*,
1975). Light–heavy bridge links position (c)
of the C_L domain to position (e) in the C_H1
domain of all immunoglobulins shown in
Figure 8, except human and mouse IgG1,
which have the L chain attached to position
(c) of the C_H1 domain. IgG has inter-γ-chain
bridges in the extra-domain region (Figure
10). Rabbit IgG has an additional intra-
chain bridge (d) in the C_H1 domain. IgM has
an inter-μ-chain bridge at position (c) in the
$C_\mu2$ domain. A bridge at (f) in the $C_\mu3$
domain of human IgM is probably inter-
subunit but absent in mouse IgM. IgE has an
additional intra-chain bridge at (d) in the $C_\varepsilon1$
domain, and inter-ε-chain bridges at (c) and
(e) in the $C_\varepsilon2$ domain. IgA has several bridges
in the hinge region (Figure 10). In the $C_\alpha1$
domain there is an additional intra-chain
bridge at (g). In the $C_\alpha2$ domain there are
probably inter-α-chain bridges at positions
(a, f, and h) and an additional intra-chain
bridge at (b)

but not in the $C_\alpha2$ domain (column 78, Figure 8; Figure 11). There are also sites in
b3/$C_\mu1$, fy3/$C_\mu2$, fx3/$C_\mu3$, b1/$C_\varepsilon1$, b3/$C_\varepsilon1$, fy3/$C_\varepsilon1$, fy1/$C_\varepsilon2$, fy1/$C_\varepsilon3$, and fx2/$C_\alpha2$
(Figure 11). All these sites are at positions analogous to those which point away
from the domain interior in the model of Fab′ (NEW). This provides further
support for the concept that all C domains have similar peptide-chain folding
since oligosaccharide would be excluded from the essentially hydrophobic
interior of the domain. The role of this oligosaccharide is uncertain but some of it
may influence domain interaction as discussed in the next section. It should be
noted that IgA is unique in having *O*-linked carbohydrate in a non-domain
region analogous to the hinge region of IgG (see Figure 10).

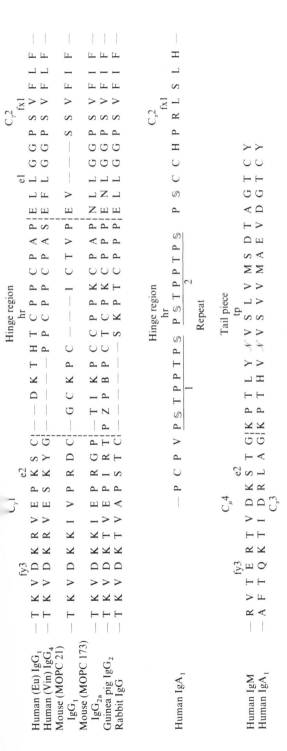

Figure 10 Extra-domain regions. The top part of the figure shows the hinge regions of the immunoglobulins given in Figure 8. Probable end of the $C_\gamma 1$ domain and the most probable beginning of the $C_\gamma 2$ domain are indicated by vertical broken lines. The centre of the figure gives the hinge region of IgA1. The first cysteine ($C_\gamma 2$) residue most probably lies at the end of the $C_\alpha 1$ domain. The unique nature of this hinge region makes the location of the beginning of the $C_\alpha 2$ domain uncertain. However, the first proline (P) residue uncertain. However, the first β-pleated segment (fx1) probably starts at the last proline shown. $\S$ sites for simple O-linked carbohydrate. The bottom of the figure shows the extra tail piece which is found only in μ and α chains. In IgM pentamers, and IgA dimers and tetramers one J chain per polymer is attached to the cyteine residue of a tail piece. $\mathcal{N}$, Sites of N-linked oligosaccharide

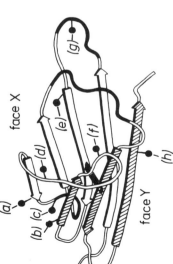

Figure 11 Sites of attachment of oligosaccharide on the three-dimensional model (adapted from Edmundson et al., 1975) of the C domain (see also Figure 6). IgG has site (c) in the $C_\gamma 2$ domain. IgM has site (f) in the $C_\mu 1$ domain; (h) in $C_\mu 2$; (a) and (c) in $C_\mu 3$. IgE has sites (g), (d), and (h) in $C_\epsilon 1$; (b) in $C_\epsilon 2$; (b) and (c) in $C_\epsilon 3$. IgA has site (e) in $C_\alpha 2$ and also sites in the hinge region

7 DOMAIN INTERACTIONS

7.1 Pairing

The high resolution crystallographic results for Fab' (NEW) (Poljak et al., 1973), Bence–Jones dimer (Schiffer et al., 1973), mouse Fab (Segal et al., 1974), and V-region dimer (Epp et al., 1974) have revealed that V domains and C domains pair at different faces (Figures 3 and 5). Contact between V domains involves segments fy1, fy2, fy3, and part of the extra loop, whereas contact between C domains involves segments fx1, fx2, and fx3. Some of the residues most likely to provide contacts between C_L and $C_\gamma 1$ domains lie in columns 9, 11, 29, 31, and 69 of C_L, and columns 7, 9, 11, 31, 69, and 72 of $C_\gamma 1$ (Figure 8). Residues in columns 11, 29, 31, 69, 86, and 88 of provide important contacts between the C_L domains in the λ dimer (Edmundson et al., 1975).

It will be seen from Figure 8 that many of the columns containing the contact residues for the $C_\gamma 1$ and C_L domains display noticeably conserved features, such as an aromatic residue in column 9, phenylalanine (F) or leucine (L) residues in column 11, and valine (V) or leucine (L) residues in column 31. Although this suggests that other C domains interact in a similar manner to that of the $C_\gamma 1$ and C_L domains of Fab' (NEW) (Fab–C-like pairing), Beale and Feinstein (1976) have pointed out that $C_\gamma 2$, $C_\alpha 2$, $C_\mu 3$, and $C_\varepsilon 3$ domains are highly unlikely to undergo such pairing. In Fab–C-type pairing, domains are crossed in such a way as to allow their C-terminal regions to come relatively close together, often linked by a disulphide bridge, but their N-terminal regions are more remote from each other. The restriction imposed by the disulphide-bridged hinge region at the N-terminus of $C_\gamma 2$ domains makes Fab–C-like pairing virtually impossible. $C_\alpha 2$ domains probably have an inter-α-chain bridge at their N-terminal ends again making Fab–C-like pairing of these domains impossible. Similarly, the inter-chain disulphide bridge at the C-terminal ends of the $C_\mu 2$ domains (almost certainly paired Fab–C-like) means that the N-termini of the $C_\mu 3$ domains must be held too close together to allow similar pairing of these domains. Likewise, the inter-chain disulphide bridge at the C-terminal ends of the $C_\varepsilon 2$ domain would not allow such pairing of $C_\varepsilon 3$ domains.

Beale and Feinstein (1976) have further pointed out that, since $C_\gamma 2$, $C_\alpha 2$, $C_\mu 3$, and $C_\varepsilon 3$ are much more closely related to other C domains than to V domains, V-like pairing of these C domains is as unlikely as Fab–C-like pairing. They also suggest that there is no apparent reason why $C_\gamma 3$, $C_\alpha 3$, $C_\mu 4$, and $C_\varepsilon 4$ domains should not pair in a Fab–C-like manner.

The crystallographic results for a human IgG Fc fragment obtained by Deisenhofer et al., (1976) and discussed by Huber et al., (1976) support the above predictions concerning domain pairing. The results show that $C_\gamma 3$ domains pair in a similar manner to the C_L and $C_H 1$ domains of Fab' (NEW) and mouse Fab, whereas the $C_\gamma 2$ domains are not in contact with each other (see Figures 6 and 14).

Deisenhofer et al. (1976) and Huber et al. (1976) have reported the introduction of a polar group in the $C_\gamma 2$ domain at a site which carries a hydrophobic contact residue in $C_\gamma 1$ and $C_\gamma 3$ domains. Such a modification could prevent Fab–C-like pairing of $C_\gamma 2$ domains. These authors also state that the oligosaccharide of the $C_\gamma 2$ domain appears to obscure some of the residues that might be expected to make inter-domain contact (columns 9, 11, 31, and 33, Figure 8). It is intriguing to speculate whether the role of this oligosaccharide is to prevent the formation of such contacts during chain assembly. The homologous oligosaccharide in $C_\mu 3$ and $C_\varepsilon 3$ domains may indicate a similar arrangement of these domains to that of the $C_\gamma 2$ domains, although the $C_\alpha 2$ domain does not have this homologous oligosaccharide site (c), but has a unique site (e) at which the oligosaccharide could play a similar role (see Figure 11).

7.2 Longitudinal Contact

The high resolution crystallographic results of Fab′ (NEW), Bence–Jones dimer and mouse Fab (Poljak *et al.*, 1973; Schiffer *et al.*, 1973; Segal *et al.*, 1974) show that there is limited longitudinal contact between V_L and C_L, and between V_H and $C_H 1$. In the model of Fab′ (NEW) (Poljak *et al.*, 1973, 1974) only segment b4 of the C_L domain is near the V_L domain (see Figure 4) and only segments b2 and b6 of $C_H 1$ approach the V_H domain. Due to the angle between the pseudo two-fold axes of rotation for the V-domain pair and the C-domain pair, V_L and C_L are more separated than are V_H and $C_H 1$. In crystals of IgG (Kol), the domains of the Fab region are arranged more symmetrically than in Fab′ (NEW) and mouse Fab, and neither V domain is in close contact with a C domain (Colman *et al.*, 1976; Huber *et al.*, 1976).

In the crystallographic Fc fragment (Deisenhofer *et al.*, 1976; Huber *et al.*, 1976), segments b1 and b5 of $C_\gamma 2$, and b2/fy1 and b6 of $C_\gamma 3$ provide longitudinal contacts. Huber *et al.* (1976) have pointed out that the $C_\gamma 2$–$C_\gamma 3$ contact is homologous to the V_H–$C_H 1$ contact in Fab crystals. In Fc crystals, there is a true axis of two-fold rotational symmetry so that these contacts are identical in both chains.

Such longitudinal contacts are important to any theory of immunoglobulin function involving changes in domain interactions and this aspect will be discussed more fully in a later section (see Section 9).

8 MODEL BUILDING

It has been shown, in the case of IgM, that data of the type discussed so far together with electron micrographs of IgM molecules free and attached to particulate antigens can be used to build a satisfactory model of this immunoglobulin (Feinstein, 1974; Beale and Feinstein, 1976; Feinstein *et al.*, 1976). The general principles which have been used are equally applicable to other immunoglobulin classes, and can be briefly summarized.

(*i*) As has been seen, on the basis of sequence homologies shown in Figure 8, it is reasonable to assume that the positions of cysteine residues may be mapped spacially onto the immunoglobulin fold (Figure 9). Inter-domain disulphide

286

bridges then provide useful clues to the spacial relationship of the domains involved, and will stabilize weak specific interactions. Where crystallographic data reveal adaptations in the folding of a particular domain, these should, of course, be incorporated when considering that of any evidently homologous domain in other immunoglobulin classes or subclasses.

(*ii*) The assumption has been made that longitudinal interactions between heavy chain domains, approximating to those seen in crystals of Fab fragments, would be conserved and used elsewhere along heavy chains, resulting in a zig-zag or helical arrangement of domains along the chain. Deisenhofer *et al.* (1976) have since shown that there is indeed such a homologous longitudinal interaction

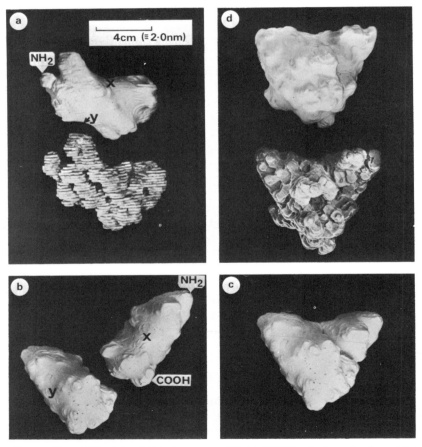

Figure 12 (a) Models of $C_\gamma 1$ domains of Fab' (NEW). *Bottom* glued wooden sections representing density at 0·1 nm intervals. *Top* plaster of Paris cast of the wooden model. (b) Two $C_\gamma 1$ domain casts orientated to give an 'exploded view' of a Fab–C-like pair. (c) Model showing Fab–C-like pairing of two $C_\gamma 1$ domains. (d) Models of C_L–$C_\gamma 1$ pairs of Fab' (NEW). *Bottom* glued wooden sections representing density at 0·1 mn intervals. *Top* plaster of Paris cast of the wooden model (seen from a slightly different aspect to that in c)

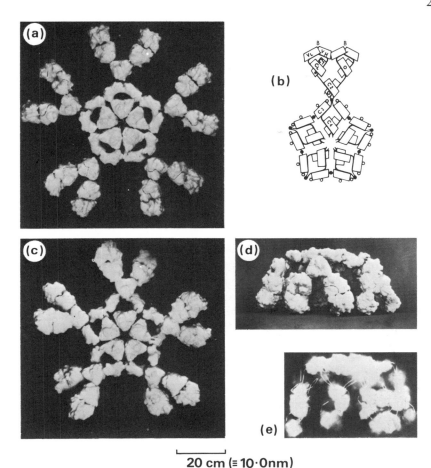

20 cm (≡ 10·0nm)

Figure 13 IgM models. (a) Model made from cast domains showing all five F(ab')₂ arms; (b) model showing only one of the five F(ab')₂ arms (from Feinstein, 1974). ●, interchain disulphide bridge; 0, site of attachment of oligosaccharide; □, regions of polypeptide chains folded into domains. $C_\mu 2$ and $C_\mu 4$ each form Fab–C-like pairs. (c) the arrangement of the $C_\mu 3$ domains modified to resemble the arrangement of $C_\gamma 2$ domains of the Fc of IgG as described by Deisenhofer *et al.* (1976) and Huber *et al.* (1976). (d) 'Table' form of the IgM model corresponding to the 'staple' in electron micrographs (see Figure 16). (e) X-ray photograph in the 'table' form to simulate the 'staple' in electron micrographs

between the $C_\gamma 2$ and $C_\gamma 3$ domains in human IgG Fc crystals (see Figures 6 and 14).

(*iii*) Where the contact residues permit it, it has been assumed that corresponding C domains along adjacent heavy chains will pair off laterally in a Fab–C-like manner. Two such pairs cannot occur sequentially along the chains without disrupting the longitudinal interactions, and moreover would require additional sequences between domains.

In the case of IgM, the model must be consistent with the electron micrographs. These will be discussed later (Figure 16). As previously described (Beale and Feinstein, 1976; Feinstein *et al.*, 1976) wooden models based on α-carbon coordinates provided by Dr. R. Poljak, were constructed of a single $C_\gamma 1$ domain (Figure 12a), a $C_L–C_\gamma 1$ pair (Figure 12d), and a $V_L–V_H$ pair, then moulds were prepared, and multiple identical plaster of Paris casts were made. Regions representing the few residues at the end of domains were replaced by appropriate lengths of wire. Figure 13a shows the assembled IgM model. As indicated in the corresponding diagram (Figure 13b), it was assumed that the $C_\mu 2$ and $C_\mu 4$ domains each form Fab–C-like pairs. The similarity of the arrangement of domains $C_\mu 3$ and $C_\mu 4$ arrived at in each subunit to those found by Huber *et al.* (1976) in the Fc of IgG was encouraging, and in Figure 13c the $C_\mu 3$ domains have been rearranged slightly to resemble the corresponding $C_\gamma 2$ arrangement more closely.

The Fab–C-like pairing of $C_\mu 2$ domains is in accordance with the frequent appearance of a compact region lying between a pair of Fab arms and the central Fc disc in electron micrographs. Although there is no stable interaction between the $C_\mu 2$ domain in isolated Fab′ fragments a weak interaction may be stabilized by the disulphide bridge linking the C-terminal ends of these domains, and possibly by longitudinal interactions between the $C_\mu 2$ and $C_\mu 3$ domains. Evidence for such interaction in human IgM is provided by the failure to observe non-covalent interactions in reduced Fc_μ preparations (Hester *et al.*, 1975) whereas the two halves of a reduced IgM subunit continue to interact non-covalently.

The arrangement of the Fab arms also was chosen to conform to the appearance in electron micrographs, where there is a considerable degree of uniformity in the angle between pairs of Fab units (see for example Figure 16; Parkhouse *et al.*, 1970; Feinstein *et al.*, 1971). This suggests a longitudinal interaction, and once again the relation of the $C_\mu 1$ to $C_\mu 2$ domains chosen to fit electron micrographs was found to resemble that between $C_\gamma 2$ and $C_\gamma 3$ domains (Deisenhofer *et al.*, 1976; Huber *et al.* 1976). Thus, homologous longitudinal interactions are used in the IgM model throughout the μ chains.

The inter-subunit bridges linking the $C_\mu 3$ domains in human IgM (Beale and Feinstein, 1969, 1970; Miekka and Deutsch, 1970) are incorporated into the model, and presumably stabilize a weak specific interaction between $C_\mu 3$ domains in neighbouring subunits. These inter-subunit bridges have not been detected in mouse IgM (Milstein *et al.*, 1975).

The situation may vary in the case of the other immunoglobulins. The same units may be used to build the $F(ab')_2$ and Fc models discussed earlier, which were arrived at from crystallographic studies of human IgG1 and an IgG Fc fragment (Colman *et al.*, 1976; Deisenhofer *et al.*, 1976; Huber *et al.*, 1976). Although the conformation of the IgG molecule in solution is not known, a possible arrangement of the units and the hinge region is shown in Figure 14. The sequence and disulphide bridges in IgE are compatible with the domains in this immunoglobulin having an arrangement which resembles a subunit in the IgM pentamer. This has been discussed more fully by Beale and Feinstein (1976).

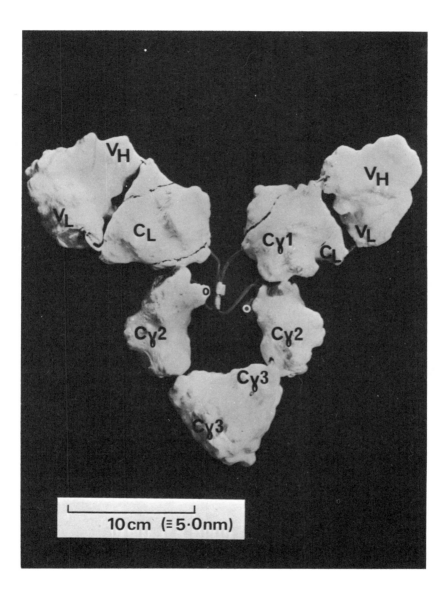

Figure 14 Plaster of Paris model of human IgG1, based on the data of Colman *et al.* (1976) and Deisenhofer *et al.* (1976) In the right-hand Fab the pseudo two-fold axes of rotation for the V domains and C domains have been aligned in the manner seen by Colman *et al.* (1976). in an IgG (Kol) crystal. In crystals of Fab fragments, the pseudo axes are at approximately 130° to each other so that the longitudinal contact between V_H and C_H1 is different from that between V_L and C_L. $\bigcirc$, sites of attachment of oligosaccharide to segment b4 of $C_\gamma2$ domains (see Figures 6 and 11)

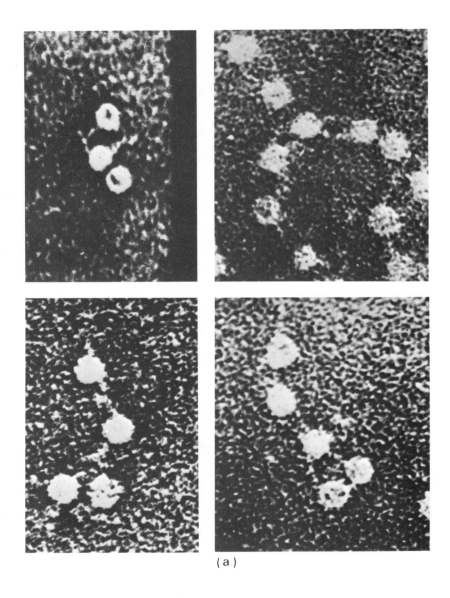

(a)

Figure 15 Electron micrographs of IgG antibody. (a) Complexes of IgG and F(ab')₂ antibody and ferritin. The angle between the Fab arms is variable. The Fc can be distinguished in the IgG complexes (left hand pictures). Note cyclic oligomers. (b) The various, almost symmetrical shapes formed by polymers of IgG complexed with a divalent hapten. A, dimers; B, trimers; C, tetramers; and D, pentamer. The Fc can be seen as a projection on most of the corners. Reproduced from Valentine (1967)

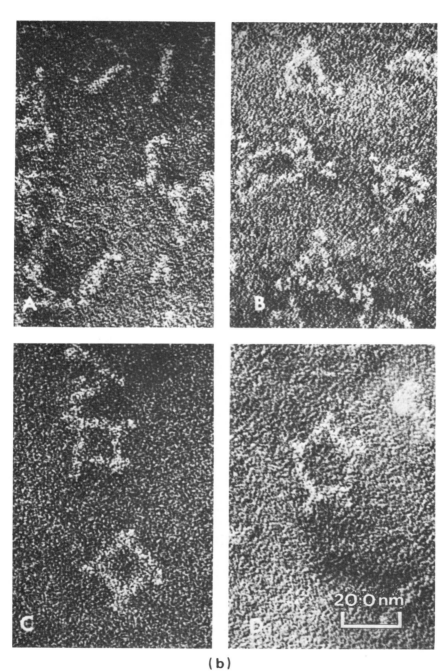

(b)

There are many explanations for IgA forming dimers in preference to larger cyclic oligomers (see Figure 19). Disulphide bridges link the $C_\alpha2$ domains just below the hinge region, which would bring these domains together in a manner quite unlike the $C_\gamma2$ domains. The $C_\alpha2$ domains lack the oligosaccharide found in segment b4 of other immunoglobulins (see Figure 11) which might prevent them from approaching each other. It may be that this different arrangement of the $C_\alpha2$ domains prevents any interaction between $C_\alpha2$ domains of neighbouring subunits of the type suggested in the IgM model for the $C_\mu3$ domains. Alternatively, the sequence differences, or the oligosaccharide attached to $C_\alpha2$ domains, but not to $C_\mu3$, near the region forming the inter-$C_\mu3$ contact (Figure 11) may not permit such interactions.

9 ELECTRON MICROSCOPY OF ANTIBODIES LINKED TO ANTIGENS

Crystallographic studies have established the general nature of the binding site formed by the hypervariable regions of the variable domains of immunoglobulins (Davies et al., 1975a, b; Poljak, 1975a, b). There is no direct evidence in favour of a change in shape of this region of the antibody on binding with antigen (Metzger, 1974). Electron microscopy has proved of some value in studying the gross conformation of immunoglobulins; early work in this field has been reviewed by Green (1969). The types of structure, seen using electron microscopy, usually using negative staining, will be examined below when antibodies are complexed with antigen in such a manner so as to form cyclic, cross-linked, or lattice structures. How these structures may be explained in terms of antibody models formed from domains linked in the manner described in Section 8 of this chapter will also be considered.

9.1 Immunoglobulin G

Electron microscopy of IgG anti-ferritin–ferritin complexes (Figure 15a) shows that there is a marked tendency to form cyclic structures (Feinstein and Rowe, 1965). In the presence of a mild excess of antigen, not only are two ferritin molecules observed linked by two or more IgG molecules, but also larger cyclic structures have been noted which show a variable angle between the Fab arms of the antibody molecules. At approximately equivalence, in larger complexes, many more IgG molecules are observed whose overall length and appearance suggest angles approaching 180°. Exact angles have not been calculated since the orientation of the antibody molecules is unknown. Valentine and Green (1967) used a bivalent hapten to obtain cyclic antibody–hapten complexes (Figure 15b). Polygonal rings containing any number from three to 10, or more, of distinct IgG molecules were seen. Some dimers and linear polymers also were formed. The angle between the Fab arms varied from 10° in dimers to 180° in some of the large rings and open-chain polymers. However, the rings were seen lying flat on the substrate and it is not known how they are folded in solution.

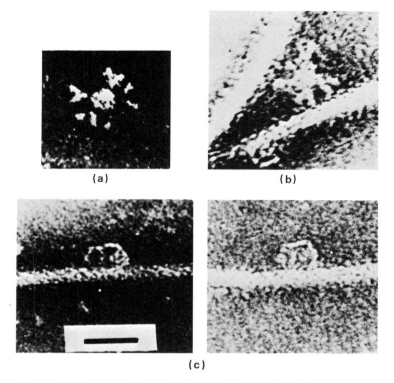

(a) (b)

(c)

Figure 16 Electron micrographs of IgM antibodies. The bar represents 25 nm. (a) Unbound IgM; (b) IgM cross-linking two bacterial flagella; and (c) two examples of IgM, seen in profile as a 'staple', bound to a single flagellum

These electron micrographs are all interpretable in terms of the domain model of IgG (Figure 14). They indicate that there is flexibility at the hinge region of the IgG molecule, but they do not reveal if there is some flexibility or longitudinal interaction within Fab or Fc units.

9.2 Immunoglobulin M

Electron micrographs of IgM agglutinating *Salmonella* (Feinstein and Munn, 1969; Feinstein *et al.*, 1971) can be interpreted as indicating only a change in spatial relationship between relatively rigid F(ab')$_2$ and (Fc)$_5$ units which are not altered visibly. In Figure 16b, an IgM molecule may be seen cross-linking flagella, or attached, with Fab arms folded down, to a single flagellum (Figure 16c) giving a characteristic 'staple' appearance. The interpretation of these pictures is that the central (Fc)$_5$ discs of the IgM molecules are seen in profile and parallel to the flagellar surface. The negative staining techniques used in these experiments do not permit face-on views of attached IgM to be visualized.

Micrographs which can be interpreted as showing similar structures have been

294

obtained for IgM attached to fragments of erythrocyte membrane (Humphrey and Dourmashkin, 1965). Similar views of IgM attached to T2 bacteriophage sheaths also have been observed.

Electron micrographs of (Fc)₅ preparations (Figure 17) reveal the presence of discs and rods. The latter structures are presumably the disc-like fragment seen in profile (Feinstein *et al.*, 1976).

Using the spray-freeze technique of Bachmann and Schmitt (1971) and of Bachmann and Schmitt-Fumian (1973) it has been possible to examine in face-view IgM molecules attached to flagella (Figure 18) (Feinstein *et al.*, 1976). Such micrographs can be interpreted as showing discs, parallel to the flagellum surface, attached through upright legs.

In many pictures of IgM, the F(ab')₂ arms appear to maintain a fixed inter-Fab angle and behave as one unit. Frequently, it is clear that only one of the component Fab units is attached to a flagellum. Various workers have shown that the pentameric molecule has an apparent valency of only five with large antigens, but has the expected value of 10 with smaller antigens, or when subunits or Fab fragments of IgM are examined. These results have been reviewed by Edberg *et al.* (1972), who showed that the apparent valency of IgM anti-dextran varied with the increasing molecular weight of the antigen from 10 through five to as low as 2·3. Values of less than 10 clearly are due to steric hindrance, which implies restricted relative movement between pairs of Fab arms in each subunit. This is in accordance with the authors' interpretation of the electron microscopic obser-

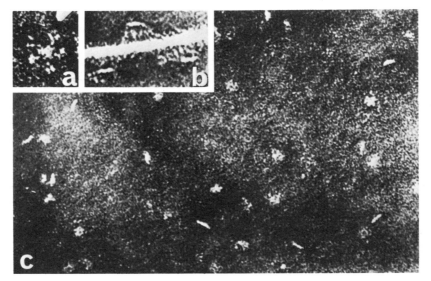

Figure 17 A comparison of electron micrographs of intact IgM and (Fc)₅ fragment. (a) Intact human IgM lying flat in the stain; (b) intact rabbit IgM seen edge on attached to bacterial flagellum; and (c) (Fc)₅ from pepsin-digested pig IgM. Similar fields have been obtained of (Fc)₅ from hot tryptic digests of pig IgM and from papain digests of human IgM

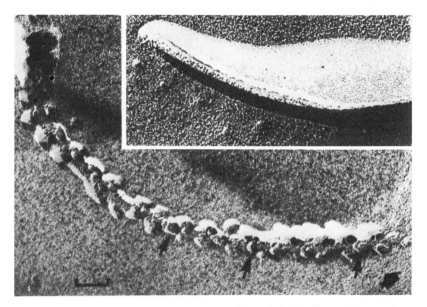

Figure 18 IgM molecules attached to bacterial flagellum. Preparations obtained by the spray-freeze etching technique were etched for 2 minutes at −100°, shadowed with platinum–carbon (in the direction of the large arrow, the shadows are white) and then backed with carbon. Some molecules seen in top view are arrowed. *Inset*, part of flagellum from control preparation without antibodies. The scale bar represents 50 nm

vations. The electron micrographs suggest a tendency for flexion to occur between $C_\mu 2$ and $C_\mu 3$ domains, although there is no amino acid sequence in this region which corresponds to that of the hinge region of IgG. A strained conformation might, however, be involved. On the basis of their studies of the depolarization of fluorescence in the nanosecond range, Holowka and Cathou (1976) claimed that, in shark IgM, the $(Fab')_2$ segments do move as a unit in this way. In horse IgM however, they believe that hindered rotation of Fab or Fab′ units independently can also occur. As stated earlier the authors believe that electron micrographs suggest little or no relative movement of Fab arms in mouse and human as well as in dogfish IgM.

When the arms of the IgM model, described in the previous section, are folded down (see Figure 13d) and examined by X-radiography, the resulting picture, when reversed (Figure 13e), simulates closely the staple appearance of attached IgM in negatively stained images (see Figure 16c).

9.3 Immunoglobulin A

Electron micrographs of IgA complexes have been the most difficult to interpret. Although primary structural information has become available

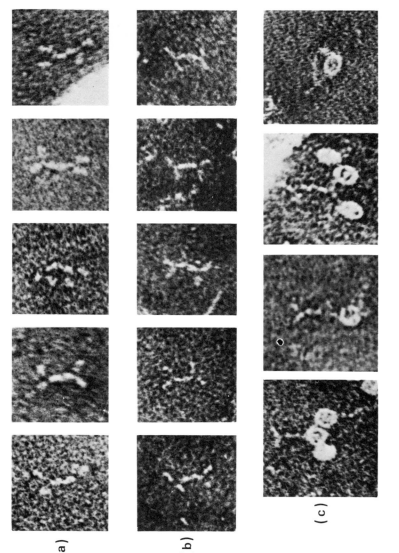

Figure 19 Electron micrographs of IgA dimer molecules. (a) Selected individual molecules of human IgA. (b) Selected molecules prepared from serum of mice carrying the plasma cell tumour MOPC 315. (c) Mouse IgA dimer attached to DNP–ferritin

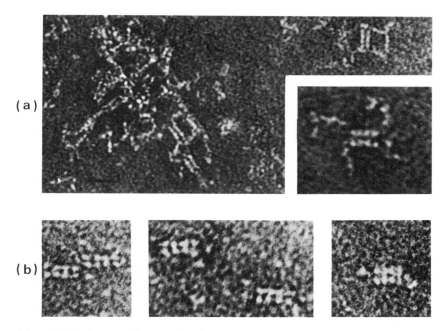

Figure 20 Electron micrographs of mouse IgA reacted with bifunctional hapten bis-DNP–glycyl-lysine. (a) Lattices of characteristic ladder-like structures made with dimer and hapten. Inset shows an individual ladder with material projecting from each of its four corners; (b) Selected individual ladders formed from IgA monomer–hapten complexes

recently, only very tentative IgA models can be devised. Unattached murine and human IgA dimers appear in double Y-forms (see Figure 19a, b).

When dimers of murine IgA anti-DNP were added to DNP–ferritin in the resulting precipitates (Figure 19c) the cross-linking double Y-shaped units appeared to be unaltered (Feinstein *et al.*, 1971; Munn *et al.*, 1971). However, using the bifunctional hapten bis-DNP–glycyl-lysine remarkable cyclic complexes of units having a ladder-like appearance were formed (Figure 20a). Monomer IgA–anti-DNP–bis-DNP hapten complexes appeared as individual ladders (Figure 20b) or as propeller-shaped structures.

Virtually identical observations have been made by Dourmashkin *et al.* (1971) who also observed double-Y shaped structures with IgA dimers, and Green *et el.* (1971), using bis-(DNP–β-alanyl)- diaminosuccinate, who obtained double bar and propeller-like images. These structures were interpreted as tetramers formed by side-by-side aggregation of two cyclic dimers of a repeating double-Y unit or, which is less likely, as a hapten-linked tetramer of four double-Y units. It was proposed that each of the four subunits seen along each bar corresponds to a pair of domains. If this is so the two Fab units in each IgA monomer have been able to interact laterally at a very low angle to each other, emphasizing their freedom of movement relative to each other.

10 POSSIBLE MECHANISMS OF COMPLEMENT FIXATION

Activation of the complement system by the classical pathway is the effector phenomenon which has been responsible mainly for speculation concerning a possible change in shape in antibodies after combination with antigens. Reid and Porter (1975) have reviewed the first steps of this process in which the C1q component is bound to the antibody molecules of an antigen–antibody complex, thereby leading to activation of protease–esterase activity in the C1s component. A feature of great interest is that different domains are involved in antigen binding and complement fixation. Antigen, as has been seen (Section 9), is bound to the V domains, thus involving the domain at the N-terminus of the heavy chain. However, complement is fixed at sites which, in both IgG and IgM molecules, lie in the C-terminal Fc region of the heavy chain.

10.1 Immunoglobulin G

There is convincing evidence that the complement-fixing site of IgG lies in the $C_\gamma 2$ domains (see Colomb and Porter, 1975; Reid and Porter, 1975; Ovary et al., 1976; Yasmeen et al., 1976). The C1q component is polymeric (Reid and Porter, 1975) and in free solution is bound weakly to several molecules of monomeric IgG with affinity constants ranging from 0.9×10^4 to $7 \times 10^4 \, M^{-1}$, depending on the subclass (Sledge and Bing, 1973; Müller-Eberhard, 1975; Hughes-Jones, 1976). Binding is much stronger (0.5×10^8—$3 \times 10^8 \, M^{-1}$ to aggregated IgG or to IgG antibody–antigen complexes (Hughes-Jones, 1976).

The attachment of at least two neighbouring IgG molecules to an erythrocyte membrane appears to be required for the activation of complement-mediated lysis (Borsos and Rapp, 1965a, b; Humphrey and Dourmashkin, 1965). Cohen (1968) found a similar requirement for the activation by IgG anti-ovalbumin–ovalbumin complexes. A possible explanation for this is that a polyvalent attachment of C1q is necessary. This could simply increase the association constant or could satisfy an activation mechanism which requires multiple attachment to sites that are relatively fixed in spatial relation to each other. No shape change of IgG antibody on binding to antigen need be involved.

After carefully reviewing the relevant data, Metzger (1974) considered that in the absence of any conclusive evidence for such shape changes, it was wisest *not* to propose mechanisms involving them. Although the authors agree with this advice, it is difficult to rule out completely the possibility of at least the partial involvement of shape changes. It is therefore worthwhile to discuss possible mechanisms in relation to immunoglobulin structure and in the light of recent crystallographic and spectroscopic results.

Feinstein and Rowe (1965) reported a variety of angles between the Fab arms in small soluble complexes of excess ferritin with rabbit anti-ferritin, when viewed using electron microscopy. They suggested flexibility about a hinge region. However, in larger insoluble complexes, formed near equivalence, the angle between the Fab arms approached 180° most frequently; it seems unlikely that the angle in these large, highly cross-linked lattices could change during their preparation for electron microscopy. Since complexes formed in antigen excess do not fix complement whereas those formed at, or near, equivalence do, it was suggested that the larger angle between the Fab arms in complexes formed near equivalence might correlate with the presence of complement-fixing sites, possibly arising from an alteration in the relationship between Fab and Fc (Feinstein and Rowe, 1965; Feinstein *et al.*, 1971). It is, however, perfectly possible the the requirement for aggregation accounts for the difference in the complement-fixing activity of such complexes.

Hyslop *et al.* (1970) prepared cyclic complexes (Figure 15b) by means of a divalent hapten, and fractionated them into different sizes. They found that monomers and dimers did not fix C1 but maximal activity occurred with rings of four to eight IgG molecules. In the inactive complexes, the angle between the Fab arms was less than 60° whereas in active ones, the angle was between 90° and 180°. The shape of the rings in solution is unknown, and again the requirement for aggregation could explain the results.

It is possible to pose a question in the negative form, and to ask if there are positions of the Fab arms that do *not* permit complement fixation? The answer appears to be that there are. Isenman *et al.* (1975) have shown that although intact IgG4 does not fix C1, the Fc fragment does so with an affinity similar to that of IgG1. They suggested that the Fab arms in IgG4 modulate the complement-fixing sites. Beale and Feinstein (1976) have pointed out that human IgG4 has fewer residues between the end of the $C_\gamma1$ domain and the first disulphide bridge of the hinge region (Figure 9) than do complement-fixing immunoglobulins. Mouse IgG1 is also non-complement-fixing and again has an unusually short hinge region (Figure 9).

A related point of interest is the effect of reduction of the inter-heavy-chain disulphide bridges in the hinge region. In rabbit IgG (Isenman *et al.*, 1975; Press, 1975) and human IgG (Isenman *et al.*, 1975), it has been shown that such reduction lowers C1 binding activity suggesting that the hinge region might be involved in the complement-fixing mechanism. However, Isenman *et al.* (1975) have found that reduction of the hinge disulphide bridges of Fc fragment does not affect its C1 fixing activity. These authors proposed that reduction of the hinge bridges in IgG might allow an interaction with Fab arms to modulate the C1-binding site. They pointed out that the possibility of IgG4 fixing the complement after interaction with antigen has never been tested, and could prove to be a genuine case of Fab arms being moved away from the modulation position.

There are two reports of complement fixation by IgG antibody—antigen complexes in which no aggregation of IgG could be detected. Goers *et al.* (1975) used the monovalent hapten nonadeca-lysyl-ε-DNP–lysine and rabbit anti-DNP antibody to form monomeric complexes. These complexes efficiently fix complement by the classical pathway. The authors suggested that although the complexes were monomeric, the amino groups of the bound antigen might function as C1 acceptor sites in addition to the site on the IgG molecule and thereby might satisfy aggregation requirements. However, these authors did not rule out the possibility of a conformational change upon binding such a large, positively charged hapten.

Pecht (1976) has reported that monomeric IgG antibody complexed to two monovalent lysozyme loops joined by a 3·5 nm spacer (bis-loop) can fix complement. Complexes with single loops (mono-loop), however, do not fix complement. Pecht (1976) suggested that in the bis-loop complexes the angle between the Fab arms of the IgG could be different from that in the mono-loop complexes.

Pecht (1976) and Schlessinger *et al.* (1975) used circular polarization of luminescence to look for conformational changes in IgG antibody when complexed to these loops. Circular polarization of luminescence is the emission analogue of the more widely used circular dichroism and is an expression of the asymmetry of the chromophore in its excited state. In immunoglobulin, the emission is due mainly to tryptophan residues, and the method is capable of detecting small changes in their asymmetry. Unfortunately such data give no indication of the nature or scale of the movements involved in these changes, but the method may be so sensitive as to detect very small changes indeed.

Spectroscopic differences were observed between Fab–mono-loop complexes and IgG–mono-loop complexes which suggests that antigen binding induces conformational changes in the Fc region. Further spectroscopic differences were observed when IgG was complexed to bis-loop suggesting additional changes in the Fc region. Reduction of inter-heavy-chain disulphide bridges removed the spectroscopic changes that had been attributed to the Fc region. Pecht (1976) argued that these results favour an allosteric change in the IgG molecule when it binds a suitably large and stable antigen, and further, that such an allosteric change may not be sufficient to trigger complement fixation which probably requires an accompanying angle change between Fab and Fc. However, the authors believe that there is no logical need to invoke allosterism, since the observed complement fixing may have been brought about by angle change alone. The circular polarization of luminescence changes observed with mono-loop binding may be irrelevant. It is important to confirm that no aggregates were present in these experiments.

In closely related studies, Jaton *et al.* (1975, 1976) used rabbit IgG anti-pneumococcal polysaccharide and a series of oligosaccharide antigens of increasing size. With oligosaccharide of up to 16 units, the complexes with antibody consist of monomers and dimers, with possibly a few trimers. These complexes do not fix complement, but luminescence measurements reveal spectroscopic differences which could be attributed to conformational changes in the Fc region of the IgG antibody. Complexes with oligosaccharide of 21 or more units contain appreciable amounts of polymer. Such complexes fix complement and show additional spectroscopic changes. Reduction of inter-heavy-chain bridges removes the changes attributed to the Fc region. These authors argue that binding of suitable antigen will induce an allosteric change in the IgG molecule but that this alone is insufficient to induce complement fixation and appropriate aggregation might be a requirement. It is felt that in this study the system is too complex to interpret usefully.

On the basis of the crystallographic results of IgG and its proteolytic fragments, discussed earlier in this chapter (see Section 3), Huber *et al.* (1976) have proposed a speculative model for an allosteric change in IgG when it binds antigen. They suggest that the molecule becomes more rigid after reaction with antigen. This is brought about through the formation of specific longitudinal contacts between domains, which are assumed to be absent in the unreacted molecule. As has been pointed out already (Section 7.2), the crystallographic results of Colman *et al.* (1976) and of Huber *et al.* (1976) show that such contacts are lacking in the Fab arms of IgG Kol, but other crystallographic results show the presence of these contacts in Fab fragments (Poljak *et al.*, 1973; Davies *et al.*, 1975a, b), Bence-Jones λ-chain dimer (Schiffer *et al.*, 1973), and Fc fragment (Deisenhofer *et al.*, 1976; Huber *et al.*, 1976).

It is thought that the allosteric mechanism proposed by Huber *et al.* (1976) as a possible requirement for complement fixation is unlikely for the following reasons.

(*i*) It is difficult to visualize how a single mechanism can be activated by a large variety of ways of fitting antigenic determinants into binding sites. (Richards *et al.*, 1975 and Chapter 2 this volume).

(*ii*) It is difficult to devise a mechanism for transmitting the proposed rigidification down individual Fab arms to the $C_\gamma2$ domains.

(*iii*) There are particularly strong reasons why it would be disadvantageous for IgG molecules bound to particulate antigens to be converted into a single specific rigid form. In cases where IgG molecules are bound to erythrocytes (Greenbury *et al.*, 1965), tobacco mosaic virus (Regenmortel and Hardie, 1976), or bacteriophage (Klinman and Karush, 1967), most of the molecules are attached to a single particle by both binding sites. A flexible IgG molecule would be essential for such double binding since the repeating antigenic determinants in different cases would be fixed in space very differently in relation to each other. On the other hand, a specifically rigid IgG molecule would have to maintain a fixed identical distance between its binding sites regardless of the antigen and would have a single fixed two-fold rotational symmetry relationship between its two binding sites. Any ancestral organism whose surface determinants fitted such rigid requirements would surely have evolved so as to evade them.

(*iv*) The polarity of repeating determinants along a particulate antigen such as bacterial flaggellum or tobacco mosaic virus particle also would be incompatible with the ability to bind doubly a symmetrically rigidified IgG molecule whose binding sites would be anti-parallel.

The specific rigidified shape chosen by Huber *et al.* (1976) is a T-shaped molecule which could not attach doubly to a surface. It would be satisfactory for lattice formation with soluble antigens and under these circumstances electron microscopy has revealed the presence of such shapes (Feinstein and Rowe, 1965; Valentine and Green, 1967). However, IgG molecules in small complexes or seen doubly attached to flagella are Y-shaped with varying angles between the Fab arms (Feinstein and Rowe, 1965; Valentine, 1967; Green, 1969).

For the above reasons, if there is a requirement for a shape change in IgG in order to fix complement, the authors would favour a non-allosteric dislocation mechanism. This could arise through the stabilization of a variety of possible final active forms of IgG differing from the inactive form.

10.2 Immunoglobulin M

It has already been pointed out that most cases of complement fixation by IgG–antigen complexes could be brought about conceivably purely by aggregation of the IgG. This cannot be so in the case of the pentameric IgM molecule, since it is known that a single attached molecule can activate the complement system (Borsos and Rapp, 1965a, b; Ishizaka et al., 1968). The IgM molecule therefore must be altered in some way when binding to the appropriate antigen.

Ishizaka et al. (1968) found that complement is not fixed by complexes of IgM with soluble blood group substances formed in the presence of excess antigen. Optimal fixation was obtained in antibody excess for IgM, but at equivalence in the case of IgG. These workers point out that their results strongly suggest that combination of IgM antibody molecules through multiple combining sites to antigenic sites on a particle or in a lattice is essential for IgM to fix complement. The formation of such complexes, of course, would involve almost certainly dislocation of Fab or $F(ab)_2$ arms. In studies which will be discussed below Pecht (1976) also showed a considerably depressed complement fixation by IgM in antigen excess.

In contrast to these results, Brown and Koshland (1975), using mono-Lac-ribonuclease and anti-Lac IgM, have reported the formation of non-aggregated antigen–antibody complexes which efficiently fix complement. Similarly, Pecht (1976), using the lysozyme loop as a monovalent antigen, has reported complement fixation by non-aggregated IgM anti-loop–mono-loop complexes. Circular polarization of luminescence studies on these complexes were interpreted as indicating a conformational change in the Fc region. Pecht (1976) argued that an allosteric change in the IgM antibody molecule is probably all that is necessary to induce complement fixation. However, he obtained a considerably lowered complement fixation in antigen excess. This observation contradicts the suggestion of an allosteric mechanism, instead it suggests that possibly aggregation of antigen is responsible for the activity observed at lower antigen levels.

It is difficult to imagine how binding of monovalent antigens by IgM can transmit a change from the V domains, through the $C_\mu 1$ and $C_\mu 2$ domains to the Fc region, unless the antigen aggregates, before or (possibly within a single IgM molecule) after binding, leading to the distortion of the molecule. It is thought that any more subtle effect normally would be disrupted completely by the gross dislocation of $F(ab')_2$ arms when IgM is multiply bound to particulate antigens, as seen in electron micrographs (Feinstein and Munn, 1969; Feinstein et al., 1971) (Figures 16c and 18). Indeed, there are cases which indicate that not every type of combination between IgM antibody and antigen is sufficient to induce complement fixation. For example, IgM anti-Rh D will agglutinate erythrocytes without fixing or activating complement (Mollison, 1972). Also, Ishizaka *et al.* (1968) and Pecht (1976) obtained little or no fixation by IgM antibody in antigen excess.

It might be thought that studies comparing the complement-fixing properties of IgM and its $(Fc)_5$ fragment could help to distinguish between mechanisms of activation of IgM involving merely the folding of Fab arms away from the Fc disc to expose sites preexisting in the Fc, and mechanisms whereby specific changes are brought about within the Fc region. Human $(Fc)_5$ preparations isolated after IgM cleavage with trypsin at or near 60° (Plaut and Tomasi, 1970) have failed consistently to fix C1 (Hurst *et al.*, 1974; Füst *et al.*, 1976; Reid, Herbert and Feinstein, unpublished observations) or C1q (Sledge and Bing, 1973) any more effectively than intact IgM. This does not rule out necessarily that IgM is inactive merely due to hindrance of sites by $(Fab')_2$ segments, since the treatment could inactivate the Fc. Moreover, a stretch of each $C_\mu 2$ domain carrying an oligosaccharide moiety which could continue to block C1 fixing sites remains on the $(Fc)_5$ disc. It is of considerable interest that $(Fc)_5$ isolated after papain cleavage of human IgM fixes C1 much more efficiently than does the original IgM (Reid, Herbert and Feinstein, unpublished observations). It is not known where in the IgM molecule the papain cleavage occurs.

In conclusion, it should be stressed that in the case of IgM, as for IgG, the authors believe that any change in antibody conformation required to induce complement fixation is brought about by dislocation of an inactive form to an active form. Such a dislocation must be compatible with a large number of ways of arranging Fab or $F(ab')_2$ arms in relation to each other and to the Fc, not to one specific conformation. The reason for making this a requirement is that each antigen will have a different spatial pattern of determinants, so that no single final arrangement of Fab or $F(ab')_2$ arms can be involved.

REFERENCES

Adetugbo, K., Poskus, E., Svasti, J., and Milstein, C. (1975). *Eur. J. Biochem.*, **56**, 503.

Bachmann, L., and Schmitt, W. W. (1971). *Proc. Nat. Acad. Sci., U.S.A.*, **68**, 2149.
Bachmann, L., and Schmitt-Fumian, W. W. (1973) In *Freeze-Etching Techniques and Applications* (Benedetti, E. L., and Favard, B., eds.), Société Francaise de Microscopie Electronique, Paris, p. 73.
Beale, D., and Feinstein, A. (1969). *Biochem. J.*, **112**, 187.
Beale, D., and Feinstein, A. (1970). *FEBS Letters*, **7**, 175.
Beale, D., and Feinstein, A. (1976). *Quart. Rev. Biophys.*, **9**, 135.
Bennich, H., and Bahr-Lindstrom, H. von (1974). *Progress in Immunology II*, Vol. X (Brent, L., and Holborow, J., eds.), North Holland Publishing Co., Amsterdam, p. 49.
Borsos, T., and Rapp, H. J. (1965a). *J. Immunol.*, **95**, 559.
Borsos, T., and Rapp, H. J. (1965b) *Science, N.Y.*, **150,** 505.
Bourgois, A., Fougereau, M., and Rocca-Serra, J. (1974). *Eur. J. Biochem.*, **43**, 423.

Brown, J. C., and Koshland, M. E. (1975). *Proc. Nat. Acad. Sci., U.S.A.*, **72**, 5111.

Capra, J. D., and Kehoe, M. J. (1975). *Adv. Immunol.* **20**, 1.
Cathou, R. E., Holowka, D. A., and Chan, L. M. (1974). In *Progress in Immunology II*, Vol. 1 (Brent, L., and Holborow, J., eds.), North Holland Publishing Co., p. 63.
Cohen, S. (1968). *J Immunol.*, **100**, 407.
Cohen, S., and Milstein, C. (1967). *Adv. Immunol.*, **7**, 1.
Cohen, S., and Porter, R. R. (1964). *Adv. Immunol.*, **4**, 287.
Colman, P. M., Deisenhofer, J., Huber, R., and Palm, W. (1976). *J. Mol. Biol.*, **100**, 257.
Colomb, M., and Porter, R. R. (1975). *Biochem. J.*, **145**, 177.
Croft, L. R. (1964). *Handbook of Protein Sequences.* Joynson-Bruvvers, Oxford.
Cunningham, B. A. (1974). In *Progress in Immunology II*, Vol. 1 (Brent, L., and Holborow, J., eds.), North Holland Publishing Co., Amsterdam, p. 5.

Davies, R. D., Padlan, E. A., and Segal, D. M. (1975a). *Ann. Rev. Biochem.*, **44**, 639.
Davies, R. D., Padlan, E. A., and Segal, D. M. (1975b). In *Contemporary Topics in Molecular Immunology, Vol. 4 (Inman, F. P., and Mandy, W. J., eds.), Plenum Press, New York, p.* 127.
Dayhoff, M. O. (1972). *Atlas of Protein Sequence and Structure*, Vol. 5, National Biomedial Research Foundation, Silver Spring.
Deisenhofer, J., Colman, P. M., Huber, R., Haupt, H., and Schwick, G. (1976). *Hoppe-Seyler's Z. Physiol. Chem.*, **357**, 435.
Dourmashkin, R. R., Virella, G., and Parkhouse, R. M. E. (1971). *J. Mol. Biol.*, **56**, 207.

Edberg, C. S., Bronson, P.-M., and Van Oss, C. J. (1972). *Immunochemistry*, **9**, 273.
Edelman, G. M., Cunningham, B. A., Gall, W. E., Gottlieb, P. D., Rutishauser, U., and Waxdal, M. J. (1969). *Proc. Nat. Acad. Sci., U.S.A.*, **63**, 78.
Edelman, G. M., and Gall, W. E. (1969). *Ann. Rev. Biochem.*, **38**, 415.
Edmundson, A. B., Ely, K. R., Abola, E. E., Schiffer, M., and Panagiotopoulos, N. (1975). *Biochemistry*, **14**, 3953.
Edmundson, A. B., Ely, K. R., Girling, R. L., Abola, E. E., Schiffer, M., and Westholm, F. A. (1974). In *Progress in Immunology II*, Vol. 1 (Brent, L., and Holborow, J., eds.), North Holland Publishing Co., Amsterdam, p. 103.
Edmundson, A. B., Schiffer, M., Ely, K. R., and Wood, M. K. (1972). *Biochemistry*, **11**, 1822.
Edmundson, A. B., Wood, M. K., Schiffer, M., Hardman, K. D., Ainsworth, C. F., Ely, K. R., and Deutsch, H. F. (1970). *J. Biol. Chem.*, **245**, 2763.
Epp, O., Colman, P., Fehlhammer, H., Bode, W. W., Schiffer, M., Huber, R., and Palm, W. (1974). *Eur. J. Biochem.*, **45**, 513.
Epp, O., Lattman, E. E., Schiffer, M., Huber, K., and Palm, W. (1975). *Biochemistry*, **14**, 4943.

Feinstein, A. (1974). In *Progress in Immunology II*, Vol. X (Brent, L., and Holborow, J., eds.), North Holland Publishing Co., Amsterdam, p. 115.
Feinstein, A., and Munn, E. A. (1969). *Nature, N.Y.*, **224**, 1307.
Feinstein, A., Munn, E. A., and Richardson, N. E. (1971). *Ann. N.Y. Acad. Sci.*, **190**, 104.
Feinstein, A., Richardson, N. E., and Munn, E. A. (1976). *Proceedings 3rd John Innes Symposium* (Markham, R. and Horne, R. W., eds.), Elsevier/North Holland Publishing Company, Amsterdam, p. 111.
Feinstein, A., and Rowe, A. J. (1965). *Nature (Lond.)*, **205**, 147.
Füst, G., Csecsi-Nagy, M., Medgyesi, G. A., Kulics, J., and Gergly, J. (1976). *Immunochemistry*, **13**, 793.

Green, N. M. (1969). *Adv. Immunol.*, **11**, 1.
Green, N. M., Dourmashkin, R. R., and Parkhouse, R. M. E. (1971). *J. Mol. Biol.*, **56**, 203.
Greenbury, C. L., Moore, D. H. and Nunn, L. A. C. (1965). *Immunology*, **8**, 420.
Goers, J. W., Schumaker, V. N., Glovsky, M. M., Rebek, J., and Müller-Eberhard, H. J. (1975). *J. Biol. Chem.*, **250**, 4918.

Hester, R. B., Mole, J. E., Schrohenloher, R. E. (1975). *J. Immunol.*, **114**, 486.
Hill, R. L., Lebovitz, H. E., Fellows, R. E., and Delaney, R. (1967). In *Gamma Globulins: Structure and Biosynthesis* (Killander, J., ed.), John Wiley and Sons, New York and London, p. 109.
Holowka, D. A., and Cathou, R. E. (1976). *Biochemistry*, **15**, 3379.
Huber, R., Deisenhofer, J., Colman, P. M., Matsushima, M., and Palm, W. (1976). *Das Immunsystem*. (Melchers, F., and Rajewsky, K., eds.). Springer Verlag, Berlin.
Hughes-Jones, N. C. (1977). *Immunology*, **32**, 191.
Humphrey, J. H. and Dourmashkin, R. R. (1965). In *Complement* (Wolstenholme, G. E. W., and Knight, J., eds.), Churchill, London, p. 175.
Hurst, M. M., Volanakis, J. E., Hester, R. B., Stroud, R. M., and Bennett, J. C. (1974). *J. Exp. Med.*, **140**, 1117.
Hyslop, N. E., Dourmashkin, R. R., Green, N. M., and Porter, R. R. (1970). *J. Exp. Med.*, **131**, 783.

Inman, F. P., and Mestecky, J. (1975). In *Contemporary Topics in Immunology*, Vol. 3 (Inman, F. P., and Mandy, W. J., eds.), Plenum Press, New York, p. 111.
Isenman, D. E., Dorrington, K. J., and Painter, R. H. (1975). *J. Immunol.*, **114**, 1726.
Ishizaka, T., Tada, T., and Ishizaka, K. (1968). *J. Immunol.*, **100**, 1145.

Jaton, J.-C., Huser, H., Braun, D. G., Givol, D., Pecht, I., and Schlessinger, J. (1975). *Biochem.*, **14**, 5312.
Jaton, J.-C., Huser, H., Riesen, W. F., Schlessinger, J., and Givol, D. (1976). *J. Immunol.*, **116**, 1363.

Kabat, E. A., and Wu, T. T. (1971). *Ann. N.Y. Acad. Sci.*, **190**, 382.
Klinman, N. R., and Karush, F. (1967). *Immunochemistry*, **4**, 387.
Koshland, M. E. (1975). *Adv. Immunol.*, **20**, 41.
Kratzin, H., Altevogt, P., Ruban, E., Kortt, A., Staroscik, K., and Hilschmann, N. (1976). *Hoppe-Seyler's Z. Physiol. Chem.*, **356**, 1337.

Low, T. L. K., Liu, V. Y., and Putnam, F. W. (1976). *Science, N.Y.*, **191**, 390.

Mestecky, J., and Schrohenloher, R. E. (1974). *Nature (Lond.)*, **249**, 650.
Metzger, H. (1974). *Adv. Immunol.*, **12**, 57.
Miekka, S. I., and Deutsch, H. F. (1970). *J. Biol. Chem.*, **245**, 5534.
Milstein, C., Adetugbo, K., Cowan, N. J., and Secher, D. S. (1974). In *Progress in Immunology II*, Vol. 1 (Brent, L., and Holborrow, J., eds.), North Holland Publishing Co., Amsterdam, p. 157.
Milstein, C. P., Richardson, N. E., Deverson, E. V., and Feinstein, A. (1975). *Biochem. J.*, **151**, 615.
Mollison, P. L. (1972). *Blood Transfusion in Clinical Medicine*, 5th ed. Blackwell, Oxford.
Müller-Eberhard, H. A. (1975). *Ann. Rev. Biochem.*, **44**, 697.
Munn, E. A., Feinstein, A., and Munro, A. J. (1971). *Nature (Lond.)*, **331**, 527.

Ovary, Z., Saluk, P. H., Quijada, L., and Lamm, M. E. (1976). *J. Immunol.*, **116**, 1265.

306

Padlan, E. O., and Davies, D. R. (1975). *Proc. Nat. Acad. Sci., U.S.A.*, **72**, 819.
Padlan, E. O., Segal, D. M., Rudikoff, S., Potter, M., Spande, T., and Davies, D. R. (1973). *Nature, New Biol.*, **245**, 165.
Parkhouse, R. M. E., Askonas, B. A., and Dourmashkin, R. R. (1970). *Immunology*, **18**, 575.
Pecht, I. (1976). In *Des Immunsystem*. (Melchers, F., and Rajewsky, K., eds.), Springer Verlag, Berlin.
Plaut, A. G., and Tomasi, T. B. (1970). *Proc. Nat. Acad. Sci., U.S.A.*, **65**, 318.
Poljak, R. J. (1975a). *Nature (Lond.)*, **256**, 373.
Poljak, R. J. (1975b). *Adv. Immunol.*, **21**, 1.
Poljak, R. J., Amzel, L. M., Avey, H. P., Becka, L. N., and Nisonoff, A. (1972). *Nature, New Biol.*, **235**, 137.
Poljak, R. J., Amzel, L. M., Avey, H. P., Chen, B. L., Phizackerley, R. P., and Saul, F. (1973). *Proc. Nat. Acad. Sci., U.S.A.*, **70**, 3305.
Poljak, R. J., Amzel, L. M., Chen, B. L., Phizackerley, R. P., and Saul, F. (1974). *Proc. Nat. Acad. Sci., U.S.A.*, **71**, 3440.
Porter, R. R. (1973). In *MTP International Review of Science, Biochemistry, Series One*, Vol. 10 (Kornberg, H. L., and Phillips, D. C., eds.), Butterworths, London, p. 159.
Press, E. M. (1975). *Biochem. J.*, **149**, 285.
Putman, F. W. (1974). In *Progress in Immunology II* Vol. 1 (Brent, L., and Holborow, J., eds.), North Holland Publishing Co., Amsterdam, p. 25.
Putman, F. W., Florent, G., Paul, C., Shinoda, T., and Shimizu, A. (1973). *Science, N.Y.*, **182**, 287.

Reid, K. B. M., and Porter, R. R. (1975). In *Contemporary Topics in Molecular Immunology*, Vol. 4 (Inman, F. P., and Mandy, W. J., eds.), Plenum Press, New York, p. 1.
Regenmortel, M. H. V. Van, and Hardie, G., (1976). *Immunochemistry*, **13**, 503.
Richards, F. F., Konigsberg, W. H., Rosenstein, R. W., and Varga, J. M. (1975). *Science, N.Y.*, **187**, 130.
Rocca-Serra, J., Milili, M., and Fougereau, M. (1975). *Eur. J. Biochem.*, **59**, 511.

Sarma, V. R., Silverton, E. W., Davies, D. R., and Terry, W. D. (1971). *J. Biol. Chem.*, **246**, 3753.
Schiffer, M., Girling, R. L., Ely, K. R., and Edmundson, A. B. (1973). *Biochemistry*, **23**, 4620.
Schlessinger, J., Steinberg, I. Z., Givol, D., Hochman, J., and Pecht, I. (1975). *Proc. Nat. Acad. Sci., U.S.A.*, **72**, 2775.
Segal, D. M., Padlan, E. A., Cohen, G. H., Rudikoff, S., Potter, M., and Davies, D. R. (1974) *Proc. Nat. Acad. Sci., U.S.A.*, **71**, 4298.
Sledge, C. R., and Bing, D. H. (1973). *J. Biol. Chem.*, **248**, 2818.

Tracy, D. E., and Cebra, J. J. (1974). *Biochemistry*, **13**, 4796.
Trischmann, T. M., and Cebra, J. J. (1974). *Biochemistry*, **13**, 4804.

Valentine, R. C. (1967). In *Gamma Globulins: Structure and Biosynthesis* (Killander, J., ed.), John Wiley & Sons, New York and London, p. 251.
Valentine, R. C., and Green, N. M. (1967). *J. Mol. Biol.* **27**, 615.

Watanabe, S., Barnikol, H. U., Horn, J., Bertram, J., and Hilschmann, N. (1973). *Hoppe-Seyler's Z. Physiol. Chem.*, **354**, 1505.

Yasmeen, D., Ellerson, J. R., Dorrington, K. J., and Painter, R. H. (1976). *J. Immunol.*, **116**, 518.